HEALTH, FOOD AND NUTRITION

HEALTH, FOOD AND NUTRITION

MAIMUN NISHA

Publications

KALPAZ PUBLICATIONS

Delhi - 110052

Health, Food and Nutrition

ISBN : 81-7835-528-0

Rs. 720

Published in 2006 in India by
Kalpaz Publications
C-30, Satyawati Nagar,
Delhi - 110052
e-mail : kalpaz@hotmail.com

Laser Typesetting at : Vinayak Printers, Delhi
Printed at : Salasar Imaging System, Delhi

THIS BOOK IS DEDICATED TO MY FATHER

MD. MIRAZ

DEDICATES

HIS LIFE TO THE BENEFITS OF OTHERS.

HE IS AS BEAUTIFUL ON THE INSIDE AS HE

IS ON THE OUTSIDE. APPRECIATE HIS

SUPPORTS ME AT EVERY SPHRE OF LIFE.

Contents

Preface

It is great pleasure to write that *Health, Food and Nutrition* will be popular among the students very soon.

Health is vital part of the great experience of living. The truth of this has been known from early times. Every age has made new discoveries about health, there by providing man with new weapons to fight diseases. Today, steady progress is being made in the field of education, nutrition, medicine, and surgery as well as public health. Attempts are being made to give every one a fair chance to lead a healthier and fuller life.

Health as a state of complete physical, mental, emotional and social well being and not merely the absence of disease. Nutrition is the science of food, the nutrients and other substances there in, their action,inter action, and balanced in relation ship to health and disease. Nutrition can also be defined as "food at work in body".

This book represents about the health, food and nutrition containing several chapters, i.e., health, hygiene, nutrition and food's role, protein, carbohydrates, energy, lipid, vitamins, minerals, water, fiber, food groups, food pyramid, dietary survey, balanced diets, planning meals, food preservation, food handling, food adulteration, metabolism of nutrients, infections and lastly nutrition deficiency diseases.

This book follows closely the curriculum prescribed by the universities in India department of Home Science and Nutrition and Dietetics.

Maimun Nisha

1
Health

Definition

"Health is a state of complete physical mental and social well being and not merely the absence of disease ore infirmity".

A healthy state of wellbeing free from disease; "physicians should be held responsible for the health of their patients".

Health can be defined negatively, as the absence of illness, functionally as the ability to cope with everyday activities, or positively, as fitness and well-being (Blaxter 1990). In any organism, health is a form of homeostasis. This is a state of balance, with inputs and outputs of energy and matter in equilibrium (allowing for growth). Health also implies good prospects for continued survival. In sentient creatures such as humans, health is a broader concept.

Concept

Health is a positive state, that means health is a state of complete well being and not just the absence of any disease. A person may not be suffering foam any disease and yet may not enjoy complete well being. These are so many times when we feel tired we are not enjoying complete well being, even through at other times we do. There are also times when we suffer from an infection ore periods of ill health. This means no person enjoys full health all the time. So we call a person healthy if he or she enjoys good health most of the time.

Sign of Good Health

(1) *Hair*. Shiny, Lustrous, healthy scalp.

(2) *Neck Glands* :- Not enlarged.

(3) *Skin*. Smooth, slightly moist good colour.

(4) *Eyes*. Bright, clear, no fatigue, no dark circles.

(5) *Lips*. Good Colour, moist.

(6) *Tongue*. Good pink colour, no lesions.

(7) *Gums*. Firm, good, pink colour, no swelling, no bleedings.

(8) *Teeth*. Straight, no crowding, no discoloration.

(9) *Abdomen*. Flat.

(10) *Legs and feet's*. No tenderness, no weakness, no swelling.

(11) *Skeleton*. No malformation.

(12) *Weight*. Normal for height, age, and well body build.

(13) *Posture*. Erect, arms and legs straight, abdomen in, chest out.

(14) *Muscles*. Well developed, firm

(15) *Nervous control*. Good power of concentration, not irritable, restless.

(16) *Appetite*. Good

(17) *Digestion and Absorption*. Normal, timely.

(18) *Sleep*. Good Sound.

(19) *Stool*. Normal.

(20) *Activity*. Heavy.

There are the some signs where body a person in good physical health.

Mental Health Implies

- Freedom from internal conflicts.
- No consistent tendency to condemn or pity oneself.
- A good capacity to adjust to situation and people.
- Sensivity to the emotional needs of others.

- Capacity to deal with other individual with consideration and courtesy.
- Very good control over one's own emotions without constantly giving in to strong feelings fear, jealousy, anger or guilty.

Nutrition is closely related with health. If a person eats the right kind of foods in the required amounts, he or she will keep good health provided no other factors intervene.

On the other hand, a poor eating pattern are eating too little or too much will result in poor health. So food is one of the crucial elements of ensuring good health. The food eaten must not only be nutritious but it must be whole-some and clean and free from harmful germs. If this is not so, the person eating the food would get ill even if the food is nutritious.

Good health is a vital part of living health provide man an instrument to right disease. But nowadays steady progress is made in field of education, medicine, surgery as well as public health. Health is a matter which effect not only each individual but also the community in which we live. An individual keeps fit, he can not make full use of his life nor can ailing community play its proper role in the world. Concept of health is vitally important to all of us and perfect health for community. To achieve this adequate food in necessity of health.

Continuously, day and night the different parts of our body are working as machine. If these go on working smoothly, so the body is to be healthy. If, this natural and normal state in upset on something goes wrong with any function of body, then body become ill.

According to world health organization (W.H.O.) health as "a state of complete physical, mental and social well being and not merely the absence of disease or infirmity".

Dimensions of Health

There are so many factors affecting health, for both the individual and the community. Ill health and unhappiness it

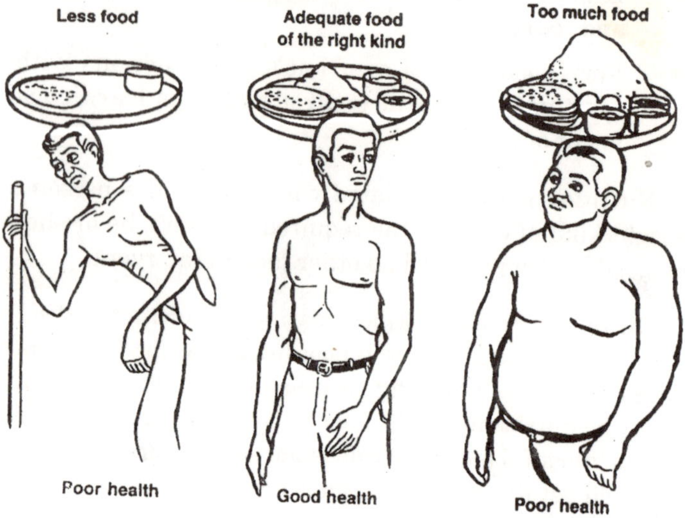

Inter-relation between Health and Nutrition.

causes can be controlled and even prevented. The following factors affect the maintenance of good health.

(i) **Physical.** This means the correct use of the body mechanism at energy stage of life, it means physical fitness. It can be brought about by eating the right kind of food in sufficient quantities along with an adequate amount of exercises and attention to the rules of health.

(ii) **Mental and Emotional.** A mentally unsound person develops physical trouble because mind and body are closely relation. Mental health influenced by emotions like, fear, agar, worry, joy and hatred ness. On the other hand, when the mind is happy, good food is appreciated.

(iii) **Social.** Social factor depends upon its progress, broad mind ness, consideration, thoughtfulness, and sympathy towards other. It influence education, productivity, health and social security.

(iv) **Spiritual.** Due to stress and stretch of modern life, is very important to consider this dimension of health. Attention to moral values, ethics, exercises and meditations are some ways of attaining spiritual factor.

Positive Health

An individual who is influenced by above this factors is in a state of complete or positive health. A person is able to live healthy in this environment and depends on the family and community as well. Food is the basic important factors toward maintaining optimum positive health. Lack of proper food causes deficiency diseases. Medicines are needed to cure or promote health and present disease.

Children and adolescents are growing and developing, and their health care needs, use of services, and outcomes are very different from those of adults. Unlike adults, children and adolescents usually are dependent on parents and others for access to care and evaluations of the quality of that care. Furthermore, adolescents differ from younger children; they are moving from childhood to adulthood and have their own unique health care needs, preferences, and patterns of use.

For these and many other reasons, a special research focus is needed to increase understanding of the issues involved in improving the delivery of health care to children and adolescents.

In 1997, six strategies for increasing the quantity and quality of child health services research (CHSR) were proposed by Christopher B. Forrest, M.D., Ph.D., of the Johns Hopkins School of Public Health, Lisa Simpson, M.B., B.Ch., Deputy Director of the Agency for Healthcare Research and Quality (AHRQ), and Carolyn Clancy, M.D., Director of AHRQ's Center for Outcomes and Effectiveness Research. In an article published in the June 11, 1997, issue of the *Journal of the American Medical Association*, they explained the need to :

1. Expand the disease orientation of health services research to include a focus on child health development.
2. Establish child-sensitive standards for setting research priorities.
3. Increase the size and capacity of the CHSR workforce.
4. Develop appropriate laboratories to study child health care.

5. Improve coordination of research funding across the Federal Government, foundations, and the private sector.

Human Body Composition

The human body comprises chemical compounds such as water, amino acids (proteins), fatty acids nucleic acids, and carbohydrates. these compounds in turn consist of elements such as carbon, hydrogen, oxygen, nitrogen, and phosphorus, and may or may not contain minerals such as calcium, iron, and zinc. minerals also ubiquitously occur in the form of salts and electrolytes, all of these chemical compounds and elements occur in various forms and combinations, both in the human body and in organisms that humans eat.

The human body must necessarily comprise those elements that humans eat and absorb into the bloodstream. The digestive system, except in the unborn fetus, is the first step in helping to make the different chemical compounds and elements in food available for the trillions of cells of the body. In the digestive process of an average adult, about seven (7) litres of liquid, known as digestive juices, exit the internal body and enter the lumen of the digestive tract. The digestive juices help break chemical bonds between ingested compounds as well as modulate the conformation and/or energetic state of the compounds/elements. Yet many compounds/elements are absorbed into the bloodstream unchanged, though the digestive process helps to release them from the matrix of the foods where they occur. Any unabsorbed matter is eliminated in the feces. Only a minimal amount of digestive juice is eliminated this way; the intestines reabsorb most of it otherwise the body would rapidly dehydrate.

Study in this field must take into careful account the state of the body before ingestion and after digestion as well as the chemical content of both the food and the waste. The specific types of compounds and elements that are absorbed by the body can be determined by comparing the waste to the food. The effect that the absorbed matter has on the body can be determined by finding the difference between the pre-ingestion state and the post-digestion state. The effect may only be discernible after an extended period of time in which all food and ingestion must be exactly regulated and all waste must be analyzed. The number of variables (e.g. 'confounding factors') involved in this type of experimentation is very high. This makes scientifically valid nutritional study very time-consuming and expensive, which accounts for why a proper science of human nutrition is rather new.

In general, eating a variety of fresh, whole (unprocessed) foods has proven hormonally and metabolically favourable compared to eating a monotonous diet based on processed foods. In particular, fresh, whole foods provide higher amounts and a more favourable balance of essential and vital nutrients per unit of energy, resulting in better management of cell growth, maintenance, and mitosis (cell division) as well as of appetite and energy balance. A generally more regular eating pattern (e.g. eating medium-sized meals every 3 to 4 hours) has also proven more hormonally and metabolically favourable than infrequent, haphazard food intake.

Role of Nutrition

The role of nutrition in health was recognized by the ancient Greeks - and probably also much earlier - who advised that food should be one's medicine. Especially Eastern cultures have for more than two thousand years used certain foods (e.g. herbs) as remedy. Clearly these early insights were based on simple observations that *nutrition* - aside from the obvious need to eat sufficient energy - has a direct effect on the health of the organism.

In the 18th century, many sailors on long journeys died from scurvy; indeed, some naval ships lost more men through illness than through enemy action. The cause of this was not understood until it was discovered that adding fresh limes to the ship's supply of preserved food seemed to boost the sailors' resistance to the illness and resulted in fewer deaths. The existence of separate compounds/elements in food that are essential for survival had been discovered, and this discovery of vitamin C which prevents scurvy spurred the search for other so-called 'essential nutrients'.

In the latter half of the 20th century, technological developments and a world-wide epidemic of lifestyle related diseases has spurred detailed research into the specific health effects of different foods. For example, in the years following the Second World War, the prevalence of heart disease in Western countries began escalating and came under the scrutiny of nutritional researchers around the world, especially in the USA. An increased intake of fat and cholesterol was thought to be a major cause, but later epidemiologic research has demonstrated that the prevalence of heart disease has continued to increase markedly despite a significant decrease in fat intake. Further, none of the performed randomized controlled trials assessing the role of dietary cholesterol or saturated fat in heart disease convincingly support the hypotheses that dietary cholesterol (unoxidized) and saturated fat (from fresh, whole foods) in and of themselves promote heart disease.

Later research has revealed the potential adverse effects on (heart) health of trans fatty acids, which were introduced to the human diet large scale with the new technology of lipid hydrogenation. Partially hydrogenated oils were added to many processed foods and helped make possible the production of solid margarine from cheap liquid vegetable oils, and helped increase the shelf-life of many foods. In the late 90's the harmful effects of excess trans fatty acids in the diet came into the attention of the public and governments began restricting or banning its use.

While one 'camp' of researchers focused on the hypothetical benefits of reduced intake of fat and cholesterol, another 'camp' emphasized the possible benefits (initially for diabetics) of reducing intake of carbohydrates and thereby preventing excess blood sugar raise and stimulation of the fundamental, all-important hormone insulin. In the early 80's, researchers began to systematically measure the amount of sugar in subjects' blood before and after consumption of foods containing a standard amount of digestible carbohydrate (e.g. 50 grams). The resulting comparable values of the blood sugar raising potential of different carbohydrate foods are ranked in the Glycemic Index. In general, the Glycemic Index demonstrates that eating processed, carbohydrate-dense foods (higher GI) results in a higher blood sugar raise and insulin release than does eating whole, unprocessed carbohydrate-containing foods (lower GI). In more recent years, researchers have focused more on the glycemic load which factors in the amount of carbohydrate eaten, whereas the glycemic index only compares the blood sugar raising potential of foods with a set amount of carbohydrate (i.e. eating large amounts of low GI foods can result in a higher blood sugar raise and insulin stimulation than eating small amounts of high GI foods).

The recent advances in molecular biology and gene technology, for example with the use of 'knock-out' animal models where specific genes are inactivated, have enabled a more informative study of how nutrition 'communicates' with our genes and thus with the chief metabolic hormones. Since the Human Genome Project was completed, the focus has shifted towards study of the proteome. The study of hormones and other cell- to-cell signalling molecules is receiving special attention.

The previous mechanistic view of food merely as fuel thus falls short. Foods and their diverse components are capable of affecting the control of metabolism directly via hormones and genes, to the effect that different foods can for example affect energy expenditure to varying degrees, also when energy intake is constant.

Nutrition and health

Ill health can be brought about by an imbalance of nutrients, producing either an excess or deficiency which in turn affects body functioning in a cumulative manner. In addition, as mentioned, the type and amount of foods we eat affect the body's hormonal environment *directly*, and a persistent intake of (a certain amount of) certain foods may induce hormonal imbalance and thereby disease. Moreover, because most nutrients are, in some way or the other, involved in cell-to-cell signalling (e.g. as building block or part of a hormone), deficiency or excess of various nutrients affects hormonal function also *indirectly*. Thus, because they largely regulate the expression of genes, hormones represent a link between nutrition and how our genes are expressed, i.e. our phenotype. The strength and nature of this link are continually under investigation, but observations especially in recent years have demonstrated a pivotal role for nutrition in hormonal activity and function and therefore in health.

Mineral and vitamin deficiency may yield symptoms of diminishing health such as goitre, scurvy, osteoporosis, weak immune system, disorders of cell metabolism, certain forms of cancer, symptoms of premature aging, and poor psychological health (including eating disorders).

As of 2005, twelve vitamins and about the same number of minerals are recognized as 'essential nutrients', meaning that they must be consumed and absorbed - or, in the case of vitamin D, alternatively synthesized via UVB radiation - to prevent deficiency symptoms and death. Certain vitamin-like substances found in foods, such as carnitine, have also been found essential to survival and health, but these are not strictly 'essential' to eat because the body can produce them from other compounds. Moreover, thousands of different phytochemicals have recently been discovered in food (particularly in fresh vegetables), which have many discovered and yet to be discovered properties including antioxidant activity. Other essential nutrients include essential amino acids, choline and the essential fatty acids.

In addition to sufficient intake, an appropriate balance of essential fatty acids - omega-3 and omega-6 fatty acids - has been discovered to be crucial for maintaining health. Both of these unique 'omega' long-chain unsaturated fatty acids are substrates for a class of eicosanoids known as prostaglandins). Alpha-linolenic acid (LNA) serves as the building block for the less-inflammatory PGE3 series of prostaglandins, whereas linoleic acid (LA) (and specifically its product, arachidonic acid, AA) serves as the building block for either the PGE1 (anti-inflammatory) or the PGE2 (pro-inflammatory) series. (The omega-6 fatty acid LA is the building block for the omega-6 fatty acid AA, but AA can also be obtained directly in the diet). The conversions of AA into the respective prostaglandins (PGE1/PGE2) have importantly been discovered to be under hormonal control, as certain hormones such as insulin and glucagon regulate the function of the enzymes responsible for the conversions. Because different types and amounts of food eaten/absorbed affect insulin, glucagon and other hormones to varying degrees, not only the amount of omega-3 versus omega-6 eaten but also the general composition of the diet is now known to determine health implications in relation to essential fatty acids, inflammation (e.g. immune function) and mitosis (i.e. cell division).

Several lines of evidence indicate lifestyle-induced insulin malfunction, referred to as insulin resistance, as a decisive factor in many disease states. Researchers have for long assumed that overfatness/obesity causes insulin resistance, which in turn causes type 2 diabetes (virtually all obese and diabetic individuals have marked insulin resistance). More recent evidence has however demonstrated that insulin resistance may well be the cause of overfatness/obesity as well as type 2 diabetes and possibly other lifestyle-related diseases. For example, it has been demonstrated that appropriate exercise, more regular food intake and reducing glycemic load all can reverse insulin resistance in overfat individuals, which means that lifestyle rather than the fact of being fat promotes insulin resistance.

Nonetheless, overfatness can unfavourably alter hormonal and metabolic status seemingly especially via the hormone leptin, and a vicious cycle may occur in which insulin/leptin resistance and overfatness aggravate one another. There is debate to what extent different dietary factors, such as intake of processed carbohydrates, total protein-, fat-, and carbohydrate intake, intake of trans fatty acids, and low intake of micronutrients, contribute to develop insulin- and leptin resistance. Most importantly, insulin- and leptin resistance are both strongly linked to chronic inflammation, which in turn is strongly linked to a variety of adverse developments such as arterial microinjuries and clot formation (i.e. heart disease) and over-expressed cell division (i.e. cancer).

A persistent high intake of processed carbohydrate-dense foods (high glycemic load) resulting in repeatedly high release of insulin and leptin seems to readily make cells less responsive to both of these crucial hormones (perhaps especially in combination with high intake of saturated fat/trans fatty acids and sedentary living). This type of negative feedback is ubiquitous in any biological system, all of which depend on appropriate hormonal regulation for survival and proper function. However, certain cell types appear to more readily become resistant to the effects of certain hormones (e.g. insulin, leptin) than others; certain fat cells (e.g. abdominal subcutaneous fat) may respond well to the fat-storing signal of insulin while other cells fail to properly receive/transduce the signal meant to induce important cellular and systemic effects. Why certain cells develop resistance to certain signalling molecules remains unclear, but it seems plausible that hormone resistance serves to protect cells from excess circulating amounts of the given hormone. Analogous to the way modern man-made pollution may potentially overwhelm the environment's ability to maintain homeostasis, the recent explosive introduction of high Glycemic Index- and processed foods into the human diet may potentially overwhelm the body's ability to maintain homeostasis and health (as evidenced by, for example, the obesity epidemic).

Antioxidants are another recent discovery. As cellular metabolism/energy production requires oxygen, potentially damaging (e.g. mutation causing) compounds known as radical oxygen species or free radicals may form. For normal cellular maintenance, growth, and division, these free radicals must be sufficiently neutralized by antioxidant compounds, such as certain vitamins (vitamin C, vitamin E, vitamin K and the aforementioned phytochemicals as well as other compounds, some of which the body itself produces. Different antioxidants are now known to function in a cooperative network, e.g. vitamin C can reactivate free radical-containing glutathione or vitamin E by accepting the free radical itself, and so on.

It is now also known that the human digestion system contains a population of a range of bacteria which are essential to digestion, and which are also affected by the food we eat. The role and significance of the intestinal bacterial flora is under investigation.

It is now commonly accepted amongst the medical profession that a diet high in fresh fruit and vegetables but low in animal fat helps to prevent heart disease and cancer.

Nutrition and Longevity

Lifespan is somehow related to the amount of food energy consumed: this was first systematically investigated in the seminal study by Weidruch, et al. (1986). A pursuit of this principle of caloric restriction followed, involving research into longevity of those who reduced their food energy intake while attempting to optimize their micronutrient intake. Perhaps not surprisingly, some people found that cutting down on food reduced their quality of life so considerably as to negate any possible advantages of lengthening their lives. However, a small set of individuals persists in the lifestyle, going so far as to monitor blood lipid levels and glucose response every few months.

This has set researchers off on a line of study which presumes that it is not low food energy consumption which increases longevity. Instead, longevity may depend on an efficient fat processing metabolism, and the consequent long term efficient functioning of our organs free from the encumbrance of accumulating fatty deposits. Thus, longevity may be related to maintained insulin sensitivity. However, several other factors including low body temperature seem to promote longevity also and it is unclear to what extent each of them contribute.

2
Hygiene

Introduction

A major chink of one's income is spending on food alone. Safe food is needed by every living organism to grow, keep healthy and have a productive life span. Food can become unfit for consumption at various stages, i.e., from harvesting, storing, cooking, serving to consuming. As such it is of utmost importance that safety of person, place and food is maintained.

Safe Food Consumption

The food handlers need to exercise utmost care with handling food for the family right from the time it is purchased, stored, cooked, processed and served.

Safety measures should be kept in mind while purchasing foods. One should keep in mind the needs of the family and the storage facilities available at home. The quantity purchased will be dependent upon the availability of money and storage space.

Buy food materials from reliable shop. This way you are assured of the cost, quality and freshness of foods purchased. It is economical to buy from super bazaars and cooperative stores. Buy from clean and hygienic stores, cooperatives and bazaars.

Some foods are eaten mean while most others are cooked. Appropriate methods of cooking ensure availability of maximum nutrients. Safe handling of food is essential to check the infection and spoilage of food during cooking and processing.

Serving of food is done by the lady of the house. At times the kitchen helpers also do this job. The health and hygiene standards of food handlers and hygiene should be high. This ensures that only safe food is consumed by the family.

Definition of Food Hygiene

Food gets contaminated when carelessly handled. The bacteria and other toxic materials may find entry into your system through improper and in sanitary handling of food. You must eat food that is free from disease carrying germs and harmful substances to keep well.

Food hygiene can be defined as "the safe handling of food in a way that will keep if safe and free from all contaminants".

Factors Affecting the Safety of Food at Home

Safety of food is a result of all the following factors put together. Any shortcoming in the functioning of one will have a direct influence, on all other factors.

(a) Cleanliness in the kitchen.

(b) Hygienic handling of food.

(c) Personal hygiene.

(a) Cleanliness in the kitchen

(i) The kitchen should be well lighted and well-ventilated. Few hours of relight in the kitchen will remain dampness besides killing some of the bacteria. A well ventilated kitchen does not smell of food odors. Insects and pests hid in dark dingy kitchen. A dry, well lighted and clean kitchen will keep insects and pest away.

(ii) Kitchen should be fly proof and hence have nest on its doors and windows.

(iii) The dustbin should have liner and be emptied out each day. Have you noticed the, dustbins lined with plastic in some eating places. The waste can be conveniently disposed of and the dustbin is easy to keep clean.

(iv) The kitchen work surface and floors should be easy to maintain and clean. Remove all food scraps immediately. It keep cockroaches and rodents away.

(v) Plenty of hot and cold water should be available for cooking, cleaning food and utensils.

(vi) Keep kitchen clothe/dusters clean. Wash them with good detergent and rinse well.

(vii) Kitchen should have a well organized storage space.

(b) Hygienic Handling of Food

(i) No dirt and disease germs get into the food she is serving to the family.

(ii) Do not leave the food uncovered. Dust, dirt and flies can spoil your food. Always use a cake cover.

(iii) If you have boils on your hands make sure you don't handle the food. Boils have staphylocoees bacteria, the toxins present in staphylocoee bacteria affect the gastro intestinal tract but do not enter the blood stream.

(iv) It is unhygienic to cough and sneeze on food. These bacteria pose health hazards and the infected food can cause sickness to all those who consume this food.

(v) It is a good practice to subject the food to visual inspection. Remove all stones twigs, worms, meevil and infested foods. Rotten and spoilt food should be discarded for safety measures.

(vi) Wash your food well to remove dirt, excessive insecticides and pesticides.

(vii) Cook food thoroughly and for sufficient time to ensure destruction of most bacteria. Pressure cooking is best.

(viii) The left over food should be stored in clean container in the fridge.

(c) Personal Hygiene

(i) Wash your hands with a good soap before and after handling food.

(ii) You should tie your hair to avoid shedding then in your food.

(iii) Tasting food with the Liddell and then returning to same cooking pot is a bad habit. So avoid it.

(iv) Avoid walking into the kitchen with dirty feet/shoes/ chappals and clothing.

(v) Sick individual should not be allowed in the kitchen.

(vi) Wear a clean apron and protect your clothing and yourself.

The Detergent in your Diet

Detergent get rid of grease and food residues from your utensils but they leave behind injurious residues.

The liquid detergents consist of soluble detergents in water. The detergent used is a sulphonate (Alpha Olefinsulphonate)-AOS the active agent is a liquid detergent makeup 15 to 20 per cent of the product.

The scouring powders contain less than 1 to 3 per cent of AOS. The scouring powders generally contain soda ash which enhances the cleaning action.

It is not easy to rid utensils of residual detergent. Since the abrasive is soluble in water, it is retained on the utensil surface along with the active detergent. Studies carried out at the industrial toxicology research center at Luck now have shown that more than 10 rinses may be needed to completely remove traces of the detergent.

A study of liquid detergent in UK suggests that 50-60 mg of the active detergent may be "eaten" by an adult each day. Babies also ingest it through feeding bottles cleaned with detergents.

Scouring powders contain proportionately less of the active ingredients. While no studies have been done on these powders—an informed estimate by experts is that the average daily consumption from them would be around long.

3
Nutrition and Food's Role

Definition

The term food refers to anything which nourishes the body, it would obviously include solids, semi solids, and liquids which can be consumed and which help to sustain, the body and keep it healthy.

The science of foods, the nutrients and other substances therein, their action, interaction, and balance in relationship to health and disease, the process by which the organism ingests, digest, absorbs, transports, ad utilizes nutrients and disposes of their and products called nutrition.

Nutritional status is the condition of health of an individual as influenced by the utilization of nutrients in his body. This can be found out only a careful and dietary history, a thorough physical examination and appropriate laboratory investigation.

Concept

Life can not be sustained without adequate nourishment Men needs adequate for growth, development and to lead an active and healthy life. Plants can manufacture the foods they need from simple chemicals derived from the soil, water and carbon dioxide of the air. Higher organism on the other hand do not possess this capacity to manufacture food from simple chemicals and hence they depend on plants or other animals for obtaining the food they need. Procuring enough food for its survival is the main aim of the life's struggle in all the higher organism.

Man has access to a wide range of foods to choose to make up his diet. All foods are not of the same quality from a nutritional needs and maintain good health depends upon the type and quantity of foodstuffs he is able to include in his diet to satisfy hunger.

Nutrition is the science of foods the nutrients and other substances therein, their action, interaction, and balance in relationship to health and disease. It can be defined as the process by which the organism ingests, digests, absorbs, transport and utilizes nutrients and disposes off their end products. Nutrition can also be defined as "food at work in the body". Nutrition must perforce be concerned with the social, economic, cultural and psychological implications of food and eating.

Nutrients are the constituents in food that must be supplied to the body in suitable amounts. These are protein, carbohydrates, fats, minerals, vitamins and water.

Nutritional status is the condition of health of an individual as influenced by the utilization of nutrients in his body. This can be found out only by a careful and dietary history, a proper and minute physical examination and appropriate laboratory investigations.

Nutritional care is the application of the science and art of Human nutrition in helping people to select and obtain food for the primary purpose of nourishing their bodes in health or in disease throughout their lines.

Good, adequate are the terms applied to that quality of nutrition in which the essential nutrients in correct amounts and balance are utilized to promote the highest level of physical and mental health throughout one's life.

Major nutritional deficiencies providing in the population and their health implications are discussed. Apart from identifying the dietary basis of these deficiencies in the population other environmental factors which contribute to the prevalence of nutritional deficiencies are indicated. Various intervention measures to the deficiencies are also mentioned. The point is made that vulnerable groups among whom nutritional deficiencies occur more frequently and to more severe degree require special attention and care.

The body requires an adequate supply of nutrients for its metabolic functions. When this is not available in the diet, deficiency diseases occur. Poor dietary intake in the most common cause of deficiency even when the diet in adequate, several factors may cause conditions of deficiency. Some of the following factors are responsible for deficiencies as follows :

- Poor absorption.
- Less from the alimentary canal.
- Excessive less of nitrogen from body.
- Poor utilization.
- Requirement of protein and fat during fever.

Calorie malnutrition is one of the most important public health problems in many developing countries including India, South East Asia and Africa. It is a wide spread deficiency disease among children of low socio economic groups. In many areas nearly half the children do not survive to the age of five years on account of protein calorie malnutrition, these who survive may suffer from impaired growth and perhaps mental retardation. The disease knows as and marasmus represent extreme form of protein calorie malnutrition. Occurs due to protein deficiency and Marasmus occur due to deficiency of calorie and protein.

Vitamin-A plays an important role in normal virgin. It is required fro proper growth of developing bony structures and health. It is needed good, healthy, moist and glossy bright cleave eyes, normal secretion of tear glands and regarded as an anti infective vitamins. Vitamin-A deficiency results in Keratomalacia, blindness, pneumonia, arthritis, acute tonsillitis, rheumatic fever among the children. Vitamin-A deficiency results in a condition known as nictalopia or blindness, night blindness, xero phthalmia, Keratomalacia, Urolithiasis etc.

Thiamine requirements of the body are proportional to the calories expenditure of the body. Normal require of thiamine is necessary. A very low intake of thiamine for a prolonged period leads to "Beri Beri" a dietary deficiency diseases. It is associated with a low calorie intake and deficiency of the other factors of vitamin-B complex that re found in foods. Deficiency is expressed as beri beri in several forum:

(a) Infantile Beri Beri.

(b) Dry Beri Beri.

(c) wet beri beri.

Vitamin B complex group is found in the body in two forum :

It is readily absorbed in small intestine but only stored in the body. Deficiency of niacin expresses itself in the form of "Pellagra". This deficiency is usually associated with a diet based on corn and adequate amount of tryptophan.

The body of an adult man contains about 9.0 gm of iron. The greater part of the iron is in the blood, the reminder in the muscle cells, other body cells and in respiratory enzymes. Iron reserve in found intra cellular in the form of protein complex as ferritim.

Iron deficiency anemia can occur all stages and among both sexes, very common among individual in under developed countries as a result of inadequate diet or poor absorption. Anemia in a condition in which there is a reduction in the total circulating hemoglobin. It is defined by W.H.O. as "a condition in which the hemoglobin content of blood is lower than normal as a result of deficiency of one or more essential nutrients regardless of the cause of such deficiency".

Iodine is a mineral compound. During the process of digestion, iodine is split from organic compounds and is absorbed as inorganic iodine. Deficiency of iodine (Hypothyroidism), endemic goitre. The iodine deficiency disease occurs in certain parts of the world where the soil has a low iodine content. Goiter is by the swelling of the thyroid gland. The reduced secretion of the thyroid controls he state of the connection tissue. Deficiency of thyroxin produced by thyroid gland, reduced the carbohydrate oxidation.

Deficiency of calcium in the diet results in retardation calcification of bones and teeth in the young. Due to the deficiency of calcium bones start bending, enlargement of ankles and wrists. Deficiency disease of calcium is called as rickets and osteomalacia in children. Repeated pregnancies coupled with dietary intake can also give rise to the deficiency of calcium.

Deficiency of phosphorus is very rare in human beings because diets having sufficient cereals. Deficiency results stiff and bones became fragile and break easily.

Every individual requires an adequate supply of nutrients in suitable proportion from growth and development.

Malnutrition can be defined as pathological absolute deficiency or excessive of one or more essential nutrients, which can manifest into over nutrition or under nutrition or imbalance.

Nutrition is the science that deals with the digestion, absorption and metabolic of food, i.e., the utilization of food in the body. It may be defined as "the science that interprets the relationship of food to the finding of living organism It includes the uptake of food, liberation of energy, elimination of wastes and all the processes of synthesis essential for maintenance, growth and reproduction. These fundamental activities and characteristic of all living organisms form the simplest to the most complex plants and animals (Pike and Brown – 1984).

Good health is a state of complete physical mental and social well being and not merely the absence of disease or infirmity.

Krehl (1956) suggested that optimum nutrition might be described as "that which provides all dietary nutrients in respect of and amount and in proper state of combination or balance, so that he organism may always meet the varied exogenous and endogenous stresses in life, whether in health or disease, with a minimal demand or strain as the body's natural homoeostatic mechanism optimum nutrition is also known as adequate nutrition or good nutrition.

Good nutrition there provides all essential nutrients in correct balance which once further utilized to promote the highest level of physical and mental health. Such a state of nutrition can be attained through balanced diets. Balanced diet not only meet our day to day nutrient requirements but also provides for an extra allowances of the nutrients to be stored in our body, which can be used in conditions of stress.

Proper nutrition therefore can not only prevent illnesses but can also remarkably after the causes of illness, when it occurs.

Nutrients :- Action, interaction and balance

The body needs each nutrient in specific amounts. Some are needed in relative large amounts and some in smaller amounts. But all are essential for our health. Each nutrient play a significant role. The mineral i.e. calcium help build strong bones and teeth. This is the action of calcium.

Teeth also contain mineral, i.e., phosphorus, both calcium and phosphorus must be supplied to the body in the required amount and proportion to ensure the growth of bones and teeth. This means normal growth of bones and teeth and maintenance of their normal structure and function requires an interaction between two nutrients.

If the diet contains too much phosphorus, it prevents the body from taking enough of calcium. Create an imbalance between calcium and phosphorus and affect the bone and teeth. This imbalance can be corrected by taking balance of nutrients.

Social, Psychological and Economic Aspects of Nutrition-Social, and Cultural of Eating

Food has a special meaning in social and cultural context from ancient vedic times. Food is the life given concept of every society. This is a desirable trend. Tolerance and adaptability to eating habits is a healthy sign of progress.

Psychology of Eating

Individual reactions to food and to the people around us can have a significant psychological influence on eating pattern.

The Economics of Food. Food casts money. It must be vitamin the reach of the people and it must be equitable distributed to all sections of the population. The availability of food and its proper distribution are of great importance.

Handling of Food and Nutrients by Body

Taking food through our mouth where it is chewed and then swallowed. It then passes down into the stomach and thereafter into a long, coiled, tube like structure called intestine. Since our body cannot utilize food as such, it alters its nature and cancels it into actions. This process called handling of food by body.

Foods and its Role

Food refers to anything which nourishes the body. It would include solids, semi solids and liquids which can be consumed and which help to sustain the body and keep healthy. Food is a basic necessity. Food is very essential because it contains substances which perform important functions in our body. These essential substances contributed by our food are called nutrients. If nutrients are not present in our food in sufficient amounts, the result is its health and in some case, even death. Food also contains many substances which are flavoring substances in food.

Food is therefore a complex mixture of different nutrients and non-nutrients can be classified into five major categories, i.e., Protein, Carbohydrates, fats, vitamins and minerals.

Function of Food

Food has three types of function

(1) Physiological function

(2) Social function

(3) Psychological function.

Physiological Function

The physiological functions performed by food over the energy giving body building, Protective and regulatory function.

We need energy every moment of our live. The energy giving function of food is basically performed by two nutrients, i.e.,

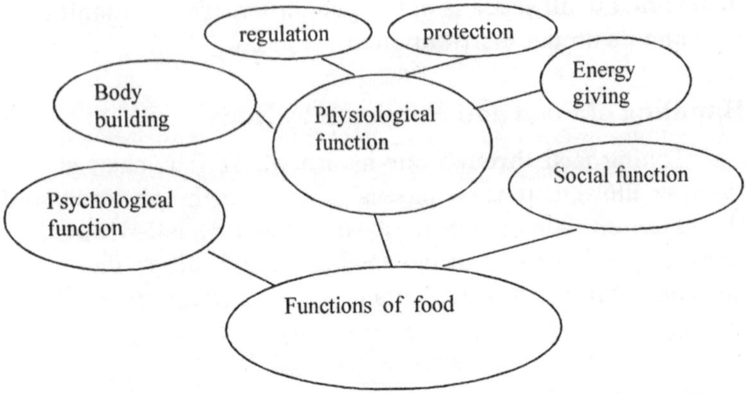

The Diagram indicates the function of food.

Carbohydrates and fats. This is why these nutrients are also referred to as the "body fuels". Carbohydrates and fats are burnt in the body to release energy.

Food is also needed for growth and repair. Body is made with of units of cells. When growth takes place, new cells are added to the existing ones. The existing ones also increase in size on the other hand cells do get worn out and die. These cells have to be replaced. This process is called repair. For both growth and repair, protein is necessary.

Protective refers to the role in providing infection by ensuring proper functioning of the body system responsible for fighting infections. If a person does develop an infection or any other type of illness, food and the nutrients it contains facilitate rapid recovery. A person eating a poor diet would take much longer to recover. He would get ill more easily as well.

Regulatory function refers to the role of food in controlling body processes. Several body processes take place in the body such as the beating of heart, maintenance of body temperature and contraction of muscles. There process is controlled vitamins, minerals, and proteins contribute substantially to both protective and regulatory functions So does water.

Several chemical reaction take place in the body, with the aid of these chemical reaction, simpler substances are used to build more complex ones complex substances are broken down into their simpler components. The rate at which these reactions proceed is carefully controlled according to the need of the body. Vitamins, minerals and proteins play a major role in controlling these reactions i.e. they act as regulators.

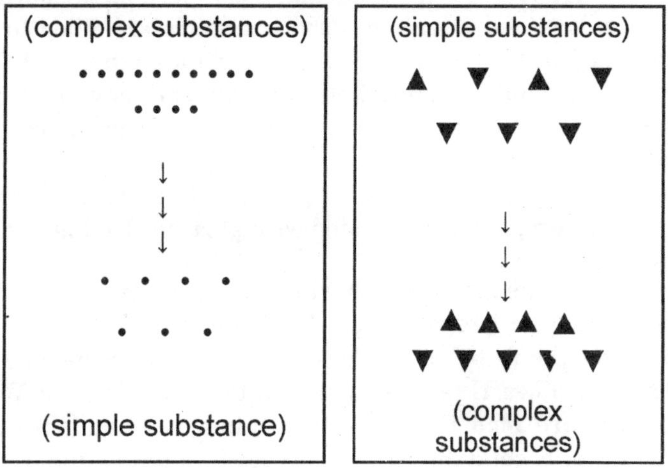

Social Function

Food also has a specific significance and meaning in he religious context. Food items such as fruits, sweets, and coconuts are offered to the deity in temples, sweets are prepared at temples and gurudwaras and distributed to devotees as a benediction or prasad. So people of a given religious community share a common eating pattern. This is because religious some foods while rejecting others. Food thus because an integral part of the social and religious life of people.

Food is an integral part of festivity anywhere in the world. Joyance occasions such as birth days, child's birth, marriage are celebrating with feast and foods. Festivals such as EID, Diwali, Holi, Dushera, Pongal, Lohri, Christmas are celebrated by special means. Food serves the function of bringing people together.

Food and eating has specific and significant meaning. Sharing food any other person implies social acceptance. When you share a meal with anyone else, you are expressing your acceptance of and friendship and respect for that person Earlier only persons enjoying equal status in society ate together. A person would never show a meal with someone inferior to him in social terms.

Psychological Function

All individuals have emotional needs such as the need for security, love and attention. Food is also closely allied to our emotions. Food serves as a reward. When a mother wishes to reward her child for doing well in a test, she may buy him a sweet on an ice cream. In this manner, that particular foods become associated with sickness such as khichree. This type of food is generally eaten. When a person suffers from fever and may, therefore, not be associated with pleasant feelings.

Food is one may through which these needs are satisfied. When a mother prepares her child's favorite dish, the child recognizes the fact that she love him enough to remember his likes and dislikes. He appreciated the attention he is given. When people share food it serves as a token of friendship and acceptance. A child quickly accepts foods eaten by his friends and by people. He admires or wants to identify with. He may even accept food he first found diet tasteful if he observes his friends enjoying its. Sharing the same food as others around him and those he considers important in his social share given him a of confidence in himself and reassumes him that he will be acted by others like him.

4
Protein

Proteins are made of amino acids, small units necessary for growth and tissue repair. Protein is the body's most plentiful substance except for water and, possibly, fat. Animal foods such as meat, fish, poultry, milk, and eggs are rich in protein. Good plant sources of protein are beans, peas, nuts, bread, and cereals.

Every single cell in your body is made up of protein. Hair and fingernails consist of fibers of protein called keratin. Collagen is the protein that strengthens your skin, blood vessels, bones and teeth. muscles are held together by the protein fibers called myosin and actin. In fact, about one-fifth of your body weight is protein. Every chemical reaction that takes place in your body - that is a lot - is dependent on proteins. These important nutrients help us build new cells and repair damaged body tissue. Because your tissues are constantly being destroyed and rebuilt, and because unlike carbohydrates your body has no means to store protein, you must make sure you get enough of this important nutrient to keep all your vital processes functioning. During digestion, large molecules of protein are broken down into smaller, simpler units called amino acids. The body requires 22 amino acids in specific patterns to make human protein and thus do its necessary functions. Your body can produce all but nine of these amino acids. The nine that can not be produced are called essential amino acids because they must be supplied by your diet. In order for your body to properly use proteins, all of the essential amino acids must be present in your system. A food that contains all the essential amino acids is called a complete protein. Examples of foods high in protein include: meats, fish, lentils, and nuts, dairy products such as cheese or yogurt and beans.

Foods are Rich in Protein

Foods are rich in protein... meats (all sorts including fish and poultry), eggs, cheese, milk, legumes and nuts. Some of these foods have more protein in them than others, and some also have more fats in them than others. meat, a food from muscle, contains a lot of protein back when you learned that muscle is full of actin and myosin in order to contract. When we eat protein, we eat macromolecules.

Role of Protein

Proteins have a myriad of functions in our bodies, including as enzymes, receptors, hormones, membrane-proteins, cytoskeleton building blocks, and structural proteins. For example, our nails and hair are mainly made up of proteins manufactured by our skin. And many hormones that have to be continually made, like insulin, are proteins. Without proteins, we would structurally and biochemical fall apart!

Composition of Protein

The building blocks of proteins are amino acids, as you recently reviewed in Unit 23. When we eat protein, we have to break it down into its amino acids for absorption in the small intestines. After amino acids are absorbed, we can then use them to synthesize the proteins that our cells need. For example, when you eat eggs, the main protein you ingest is one called ovalbumin (similar to albumin); our bodies break that down into amino acids, and then we can make keratin or enzymes or fibrinogen, or whatever we need. We can totally recycle the ovalbumin amino acids into new proteins... It's kind of like being able to disassemble a desk in order to make a chair and footstool from the parts.

Storing Protein

The cells in our bodies are constantly making and breaking down proteins. There are normal anabolic and catabolic reactions to do this. In order to build a protein you must already have most of the amino acids... that is because there are some essential amino acids that we cannot make but that we have to ingest. There are 20 amino acids that we use to make proteins, and 8 of them (10 in children) are essential amino acids. When we breakdown proteins, much of the time we can just recycle the amino acids into new proteins that we are going to make.

However, when we breakdown proteins in order to make energy, like when we haven't eaten any carbohydrates in a while, the reaction (gluconeogenesis) plucks off the nitrogen portion of the amino acids from the proteins and dumps this portion as nitrogenous waste. This nitrogenous waste is cellular waste, and is removed from our bodies by the urinary system.

Requirement of Protein for Body

Your book describes needing approximately 0.4 grams of protein per pound of body weight. Let's assume that our class average body weight is 150 pounds (I am assuming that I skew us toward a heavier than normal amount!), then that means that we each have to take in 60 grams of protein per day. Converted into ounces, that means that we only have to each take in approximately 2 ounces of protein per day!

If we put that back together with our carbohydrate amount (approximately 9 oz) and the amount of lipid we should have in a day (no more than 30 per cent of total), if we eat 15 oz of food each day, 9 oz from carbohydrates, 2 oz from protein, and 4 oz of fat, we will have taken in all that we need. I guess the reason that I because the average weight to be so high is that I hardly ever eat less than one pound of food in a day!

In addition to our need for proteins, carbohydrates, nucleic acids, and lipids in our diets, we also need some other molecules. Some of these molecules are also organic molecules, and therefore contain carbon and hydrogen atoms within them. These additional organic molecules that we need are called vitamins. Other molecules that we need in our diets are not organic, and are called minerals.

Protein need

After water, the biggest component in your body is protein. Over 98 per cent of the molecules in your body are replaced every year. So you need protein as a building block. If you don't get enough protein, or if you are eating poor quality protein, your body will not grow strong muscles, bones, blood, teeth, etc.

The *Eat Right For Your Blood Type* diet's Peter D'adamo recommends different ratios for each blood type. His rough guidelines are 20 per cent for A & AB, 34 per cent for B, and 45 per cent for O types. The metabolic diets don't specify protein requirements in grams, but *Hunter-Gatherers* need animal protein at every meal, whereas extreme *Agriculturists* thrive on a vegetarian diet.

Traditional nutritionists will probably recommend 10-15% of calories. A lot of naturopathic nutritionists are concerned that the level of protein consumption is too high. I have seen recommendations ranging from .6g/kg/day to 1g/kg/day.

Protein : Moving Closer to Center Stage

Until recently, protein got little attention. Like a quiet child in a classroom of rowdies, it was often overshadowed by fat, carbohydrates, and vitamins. That's changing. Lately there's been an explosion of interest in protein, largely triggered by high-protein diets for weight loss.

Surprisingly little is known about protein and health. We know that adults need a minimum of 1 gram of protein for every kilogram of body weight per day to keep from slowly breaking down their own tissues. That's about 9 grams of protein for every 20 pounds. Beyond that, there's relatively little solid information on the ideal amount of protein in the diet, a healthy target for calories contributed by protein, or the best kinds of protein.

Around the world, millions of people don't get enough protein. Protein malnutrition leads to the condition known as kwashiorkor. Lack of protein can cause growth failure, loss of muscle mass, decreased immunity, weakening of the heart and respiratory system, and death.

In the United States and other developed countries, getting the minimum daily requirement of protein is easy. Cereal with milk for breakfast, a peanut butter and jelly sandwich for lunch, and a piece of fish with a side of beans for dinner adds up to about 70 grams of protein, *plenty for the average adult.*

Digesting it releases acids that the body usually neutralizes with calcium and other buffering agents in the blood. Eating lots of protein, such as the amounts recommended in the so-called low-carb or no-carb diets, takes lots of calcium. Some of this may be pulled from bone. Following a high-protein diet for a few weeks probably won't have much effect on bone strength. Doing it for a long time, though, could weaken bone. In the Nurses' Health Study, for example, women who ate more than 95 grams of protein a day were 20 per cent more likely to have broken a wrist over a 12-year period when compared to those who ate an average amount of protein (less than 68 grams a day). Although more research is clearly needed to define the optimal amount of daily protein, these results suggest that long-term high-protein diets should be used with caution, if at all.

Protein : is n't Alike

Some of the protein you eat contains all the amino acids needed to build new proteins. This kind is called complete protein. Animal sources of protein tend to be complete. Other protein sources lack one or more amino acids that the body can't make from scratch or create by modifying another amino acid. Called incomplete proteins, these usually come from fruits, vegetables, grains, and nuts.

Vegetarians need to be aware of this. To get all the amino acids needed to make new protein - and thus to keep the body's systems in good shape - people who don't eat meat, fish, poultry, eggs, or dairy products should eat a variety of protein-containing foods each day.

Protein : Package

Animal protein and vegetable protein probably have the same effects on health. It's the protein package that's likely to make a difference. A 6-ounce broiled Porterhouse steak is a great source of complete protein - 38 grams worth. But it also delivers 44 grams of fat, 16 of them saturated. That's almost three-fourths of the recommended daily intake for saturated fat. The same amount of salmon gives you 34 grams of protein and 18 grams of fat, 4 of them saturated. A cup of cooked lentils has 18 grams of protein, but under 1 gram of fat.

The bottom line is that it's important to pay attention to what comes along with the protein in your food choices. If you are partial to beef, stick with the leanest cuts. Fish or poultry are excellent alternatives. Even better options are vegetable sources of protein, such as beans, nuts, and whole grains.

Protein : Chronic Disease

The most solid connection between proteins and health has to do with allergies. Proteins in food and the environment are responsible for these overreactions of the immune system to what should be harmless proteins. Beyond that, relatively little evidence has been gathered regarding the effect of protein on the development of chronic diseases.

- ***Cardiovascular disease.*** To date, only one large, prospective study - the Nurses' Health Study - has investigated the association between dietary protein and heart disease or stroke. In this study, women who ate the most protein (about 110 grams per day) were 25 percent less likely to have had a heart attack or to have died of heart disease than the women who ate the least protein (about 68 grams per day) over a 14-year period. (3) Whether the protein came from animals or vegetables or whether it was part of low-fat or higher-fat diets didn't seem to matter. These results offer reassurance that eating a lot of protein doesn't harm the heart. In fact, it is possible that eating more protein while cutting back on easily digested carbohydrates may be benefit the heart.
- ***Diabetes.*** Although proteins found in cow's milk have been implicated in the development of type 1 diabetes (formerly called juvenile or insulin-dependent diabetes), ongoing research has yielded inconsistent results. Later

in life, the amount of protein in the diet doesn't seem to adversely affect the development of type 2 (adult-onset) diabetes, although research in this area is ongoing.

- ***Cancer.*** There's no good evidence that eating a little protein or a lot of it influences cancer risk.

Protein : Weight Control

The notion that you could lose weight by cutting out carbohydrates and eating plenty of protein was once tut-tutted by the medical establishment partly because such diets were based on little more than interesting ideas and speculation. In the past two years, head-to-head trials that pitted high-protein, low-carbohydrate diets against low-fat, high-carbohydrate diets have given them a scientific leg to stand on. These trials show that high-protein, low-carbohydrate diets may work more quickly than low-fat diets, at least in the first six months. After a year or so, though, weight loss is about equal.(5-9) Compared with a low-fat, high-carbohydrate diet, a higher-protein diet that goes easy on saturated and trans fats may decrease the amount of triglycerides in the blood, which is also good for the heart.

Why do high-protein, low-carb diets seem to work more quickly than low-fat, high-carbohydrate diets? First, chicken, beef, fish, beans, or other high-protein foods slow the movement of food from the stomach to the intestine. Slower stomach emptying means you feel full for longer and get hungrier later. Second, protein's gentle, steady effect on blood sugar avoids the quick, steep rise in blood sugar and just as quick hunger-bell-ringing fall that occurs after eating a rapidly digested carbohydrate, like white bread or baked potato. Third, the body uses more energy to digest protein than it does to digest fat or carbohydrate.

There's no need to go overboard on protein and eat it to the exclusion of everything else. Avoiding fruits, vegetables, and whole grains means missing out on healthful fiber, vitamins, minerals, and other phytonutrients. It's also important to pay attention to what accompanies protein. Choosing high-protein foods that are low in saturated fat will help the heart even as it helps the waistline.

Protein : Theme

Take away the water and about 75 per cent of your weight is protein. This chemical family is found throughout the body. It's in muscle, bone, skin, hair, and virtually every other body part or tissue. It makes up the enzymes that power many chemical reactions and the hemoglobin that carries oxygen in your blood. At least 10,000 different proteins make you what you are and keep you that way.

Twenty or so basic building blocks, called amino acids, provide the raw material for all proteins. Following genetic instructions, the body strings together amino acids. Some genes call for short chains, others are blueprints for long chains that fold, origami-like, into intricate, three-dimensional structures.

Because the body doesn't store amino acids, as it does fats or carbohydrates, it needs a daily supply of amino acids to make new protein.

Nuts for the Heart

Many people think of nuts as just another junk food snack. In reality, nuts are excellent sources of protein and other healthful nutrients.

One surprising finding from nutrition research is that people who regularly eat nuts are less likely to have heart attacks or die from heart disease than those who rarely eat them. Several of the largest cohort studies, including the Adventist Study, the Iowa Women's Health Study, the Nurses' Health Study, and the Physicians' Health Study have shown a consistent 30 per cent to 50 per cent lower risk of myocardial infarction, sudden cardiac death, or cardiovascular disease associated with eating nuts several times a week. In fact, the FDA now allows some nuts and foods made with them to carry this claim: "Eating a diet that includes one ounce of nuts daily can reduce your risk of heart disease."

There are several ways that nuts could have such an effect. The unsaturated fats they contain help lower LDL (bad) cholesterol and raise HDL (good) cholesterol. One group of unsaturated fat found in walnuts, the omega-3 fatty acids, appears to prevent the development of erratic heart rhythms. Omega-3 fatty acids (which are also found in fatty fish such as salmon and bluefish) may also prevent blood clots, much as aspirin does. Nuts are rich in arginine, an amino acid needed to make a molecule called nitric oxide that relaxes constricted blood vessels and eases blood flow. They also contain vitamin E, folic acid, potassium, fiber, and other healthful nutrients.

Eating nuts won't do much good if you gobble them in addition to your usual snacks and meals. At 185 calories per ounce, a handful of walnuts a day could add 10 pounds or more in a year if you don't cut back on something else. This weight gain would tip the scales toward heart disease, not away from it. Instead, eat nuts instead of chips or other, less healthy snacks. Or try using them instead of meat in main dishes, or as a healthful crunch in salads

Talk about Soy

The U.S. Food and Drug Administration now allows food makers to claim on the label of low-fat foods containing at least 6.25 grams of soy protein that soy can help reduce the risk of heart disease.

One protein source that has been getting a lot of attention is soybeans. Some research suggests that regularly eating soy-based foods lowers cholesterol, chills hot flashes, prevents breast and prostate cancer, aids weight loss, and wards off osteoporosis. These effects may be due to a unique characteristic of soybeans-their high concentrations of is flavones, a type of plant-made estrogen.

This research has prompted scads of media reports touting the joys of soy. It also has food makers churning out new soy products that are beginning to move into the mainstream. In Boston, for example, soymilk is now advertised on the radio during Boston Red Sox games, alongside donuts, oil additives, and beer.

The U.S. Food and Drug Administration now allows food makers to claim on the labels of low-fat foods containing at least

6.25 grams of soy protein that soy can help reduce the risk of heart disease.

As is so often the case, though, many of the claims made for soy go far beyond the available evidence.

- ***Heart disease.*** There's decent evidence that soy lowers cholesterol levels. A 1995 meta-analysis of 38 controlled clinical trials showed that eating approximately 50 grams of soy protein a day in place of animal protein reduced total cholesterol levels by 9.3 per cent, LDL cholesterol by 12.9 per cent, and triglycerides by 10.5 per cent. Such reductions, if sustained over time, could mean a 20 percent reduction in the risk of heart attack, stroke, or other forms of cardiovascular disease. Individuals with very high cholesterol levels, in the vicinity of 300 mg/dL, appeared to benefit most from eating soy-based foods. Keep in mind that 50 grams of soy protein is the equivalent of 1½ pounds of tofu or eight 8-ounce glasses of soymilk a day. The American Heart Association now recommends including soy-based foods as part of a heart-healthy diet.
- ***Hot flashes.*** Soy has also been investigated as a treatment for hot flashes and other problems that often accompany menopause. In theory, this makes sense. Soybeans are rich in plant estrogens, also called phytoestrogens. In some tissues, these substances mimic the action of estrogen. So they could cool hot flashes by giving a woman an estrogen-like boost during a time of dwindling estrogen levels. Yet carefully controlled studies haven't found this to be the case.
- ***Breast cancer.*** In some tissues, phytoestrogens block the action of estrogen. If this occurs in breast tissue, for example, then eating soy could reduce the risk of breast cancer because estrogen stimulates the growth and multiplication of breast and breast cancer cells. However, studies to date haven't provided a clear answer, with some showing a benefit and others showing no association between soy consumption and breast cancer. In fact, a handful of unsettling reports suggest that concentrated supplements of soy proteins may stimulate

the growth of breast cancer cells. Large prospective studies now underway should offer better information regarding soy and breast cancer risk.

- ***Memory and thinking ability :*** A few studies have raised the possibility that eating soy could help prevent the age-related loss of memory or decline in cognitive function. Two recent trials have yielded contradictory results in this area, with one showing a benefit for soy and another showing no benefit Others go further, and suggest that too much soy could lead to memory problems. Among older women of Japanese ancestry living in Hawaii, those who relied on the traditional soy-based diet were more likely to have cognitive problems than those who switched to a more Western diet.

Recommendations for Protein Intake

- ***Get a good mix of proteins.*** Almost any reasonable diet will give you enough protein each day. Eating a variety of foods will ensure that you get all of the amino acids you need.
- ***Pay attention to the protein package.*** You rarely eat straight protein. Some comes packaged with lots of unhealthy fat, like when you eat marbled beef or drink whole milk. If you eat meat, steer yourself toward the leanest cuts. If you like dairy products, skim or low-fat versions are healthier choices. Beans, soy, nuts, and whole grains offer protein without much saturated fat and with plenty of healthful fiber and micronutrients.
- ***Balance carbohydrates and protein.*** Cutting back on highly processed carbohydrates and increasing protein improves levels of blood triglycerides and HDL, and so may reduce your chances of having a heart attack, stroke, or other form of cardiovascular disease. It may also make you feel full longer, and stave off hunger pangs. Too much protein, though, could weaken bones.
- ***Eat soy in moderation.*** Soybeans, tofu, and other soy-based foods are an excellent alternative to red meat. But don't go overboard. Two to four servings a week is a good target. And stay away from supplements that contain

concentrated soy protein or soy extracts, such as isoflavones. Larger amounts of soy may soothe hot flashes and other menopause-associated problems, but the evidence for this is weak.

Dietary Sources of Protein

Food	*Serving*	*Weight in grams*	*Protein grams*	*Daily value%*
Hamburger, extra lean	6 ounces	170	48.6	97
Chicken, roasted	6 ounces	170	42.5	85
Fish	6 ounces	170	41.2	82
Tuna, water packed	6 ounces	170	40.1	80
Beefsteak, broiled	6 ounces	170	38.6	77
Cottage cheese	1 cup	225	28.1	56
Cheese pizza	2 slices	128	15.4	31
Yogurt, low fat	8 ounces	227	11.9	24
Tofu	1/2 cup	126	10.1	20
Lentils, cooked	1/2 cup	99	9	18
Skim milk	1 cup	245	8.4	17
Split peas, cooked	1/2 cup	98	8.1	16
Whole milk	1 cup	244	8	16
Lentil soup	1 cup	242	7.8	16
Kidney beans, cooked	1/2 cup	87	7.6	15
Cheddar cheese	1 ounce	28	7.1	14
Macaroni, cooked	1 cup	140	6.8	14
Soymilk	1 cup	245	6.7	13
Egg	1 large	50	6.3	13
Whole wheat bread	2 slices	56	5.4	11
White bread	2 slices	60	4.9	10
Rice, cooked	1 cup	158	4.3	9
Broccoli, cooked	5 inch piece	140	4.2	8
Baked potato	2x5 inches	156	3	6
Corn, cooked	1 ear	77	2.6	5

5
Carbohydrates

Starches and sugars are carbohydrates, the main source of the body's energy. Carbohydrates account for about half of the calorie intake for most Americans and up to four fifths of the calories in diets of African and Asian peoples. Carbohydrate-rich foods are also the main sources of protein for most of the world. Rice, wheat, corn, and potatoes are common rich sources of carbohydrates.

Sugars are not essential foods. They provide energy (calories) but no nutrients. For that reason sugar is called an "empty calorie" food. Occasional sweets are not harmful to a healthy, active person, but excessive sugar can lead to tooth decay when eaten between meals, especially in sticky snack foods that cling to the teeth. (*See also* Carbohydrates.)

Most of our energy comes from carbohydrates. Carbohydrates are chemical compounds of carbon, hydrogen and oxygen. They provide us with calories which can be converted into energy. There are two types of carbohydrates: simple, which are sugars, or complex, which are starches. It's a good idea to try to eat more complex carbohydrates because your body get longer sustained energy from these foods. Examples of complex carbohydrates include: potatoes, pasta, bread, rice, lentils, cereals and fruits and vegetables. Compare these to the simple carbohydrates such as cookies, candy bars and other sugar foods which provide a quick jolt of energy, but then leave your body craving more. These simple carbohydrates are known as "empty calories" because they lack vitamins, minerals, fiber or anything of value to your system.

Composition of carbohydrates

Carbohydrates are polysaccharides and sugars. The most common and useful polysaccharides are starch (found only in plants) and glycogen (found mainly in muscle, or meat, and the liver). You see, when a plant has made (through photosynthesis) plenty of monosaccharide, it needs to store them for later use (like at night when it is dark outside). So the plant stores these monosaccharides (simple sugars) as starch. Meanwhile, in animals, we need the monosaccharides anywhere in our bodies where we need to make lots of ATP- and muscle is certainly a place for that! So, our muscles gather up the monosaccharides and store them as glycogen for later use. Therefore, when we look for food that is rich in polysaccharides, we typically look at foods derived from starchy plants and at meat.

Another polysaccharide that we eat is cellulose. It is the carbohydrate that makes up the cell walls of plant cells, and provides tough structure for the plants (since they lack bones). We have difficult time digesting cellulose, and, as mentioned in Unit 24, we rely on beneficial bacteria in our small intestines to get any of the monosaccharides out of cellulose. However, most of the cellulose we ingest still passes through our digestive system as unabsorbable material. Even though it is unabsorbed, it is useful in that it provides the fiber (a.k.a., roughage or bulk) in our diets that helps peristalsis of the alimentary canal to be effective.

Some disaccharides and monosaccharides in our diets. Common table sugar is a disaccharide. And anyone who has ever been around a kid after he/she has eaten a lot of sugar knows that the kid's digestive system was able to pick up a lot of sugars from that meal!

Role of Carbohydrate

Carbohydrates are used with oxygen to perform cellular respiration and produce ATP. Without carbohydrates we would run out of energy and our cells would die. Therefore, if we don't have enough available, we will make more from other molecules.

Micronutrients of Carbohydrate

Monosaccharides (or simple sugars) are the absorbable micronutrients of the carbohydrates. All monosaccharides have the same molecular formula of $C_6H_{12}O_6$. These atoms can be put together in a variety of ways, so there are multiple types of monosaccharides. The most important one is glucose, since it is vital for cellular respiration (even without oxygen it can be used to make ATP and build up lactic acid). There are other monosaccharides, like fructose and galactose, but these can be converted into glucose within liver cells in order to be more useful.

Storing carbohydrates

Glycogensis— literally, the making of glycogen. Glycogen is our storage polysaccharide for glucose, so, if we have a lot of glucose running around in our bodies, we convert it into glycogen using the chemical reactions called glycogensis.

Glycogenolysis— literally, the breakdown of glycogen. When glucose is in short supply, we breakdown any glycogen that we have (glycogen isn't typically for long-term storage).

Fluconeogenesis— when we do not have enough glucose and we have no more glycogen, we still need to make glucose available.

Carbohydrate Need

It depends on how active we are. The more active, the more carbohydrates are needed. Your book says that an average person takes in 200 - 300 grams of carbohydrates daily— of that amount, somewhere around 150 grams is absolutely necessary if you are not going to break down proteins to make your energy. Converted into ounces, 200 - 300 g is the same as approximately 7 - 10 oz. This amount is only the amount of *usable* carbohydrates that we take in each day... it does not include the roughage in our diets.

Requirement of Carbohydrate

Protein, essential fats and micronutrients are primarily used as building materials. Carbohydrate is the only nutrient whose primary role is as fuel. To get lean, we want to burn up our supplies of excess fat, but to get consistently good performance, we need to give our bodies the right kind of fuel at the right time.

During exercise, we use ATP (adenosine troposphere) which our bodies can get more easily from muscle glycogen and blood glucose than from stored fat. Muscle glycogen comes from blood glucose, which comes from the carbohydrates that we eat.

Peter D'adamo (Eat Right For Your Blood Type) recommends different ratios for each blood type. His rough guidelines are 72 per cent for A, 60 per cent for AB, 56 per cent for B, and 38 per cent for O types. The metabolic diets range from minimal carbohydrates for extreme Hunter-Gatherers to high carbohydrates for extreme Agriculturists. Traditional nutritionists and naturopaths tend to favour high carbohydrates diets.

Types of Carbohydrates

Classification based on number of sugar units in total chain.

- Monosaccharides - single sugar unit
- Disaccharides- two sugar unit
- Oligosaccharaides- 3 to 10 sugar units
- Poly saccharides morethan 10 units.

Carbohydrates Role

Carbohydrates come from a wide array of foods - bread, beans, milk, popcorn, potatoes, cookies, spaghetti, corn, and cherry pie. They also come in a variety of forms. The most common and abundant are sugars, fibers, and starches. The basic building block of a carbohydrate is a sugar molecule, a simple union of carbon, hydrogen, and oxygen. Starches and fibers are essentially chains of sugar molecules. Some contains hundreds of sugars. Some chains are straight, others branch wildly.

Carbohydrates were once grouped into two main categories. Simple carbohydrates included sugars such as fruit sugar (fructose), corn or grape sugar (dextrose or glucose), and table sugar (sucrose). Complex carbohydrates included everything made of three or more linked sugars. Simple sugars were considered bad and complex carbohydrates good. The picture is much more complicated than that.

The digestive system handles all carbohydrates in much the same way - it breaks them down (or tries to break them down) into single sugar molecules, since only these are small enough to cross into the bloodstream. It also converts most digestible carbohydrates into glucose (also known as blood sugar), because cells are designed to use this as a universal energy source.

Fiber is an exception. It is put together in such a way that it can't be broken down into sugar molecules, and so passes through the body undigested.

Carbohydrates and the Glycemic Index

A new system for classifying carbohydrates calls into question many of the old assumptions about how carbohydrates affect health. This new system, known as the glycemic index, measures how fast and how far blood sugar rises after you eat a food that contains carbohydrates.

White bread, for example, is converted almost immediately to blood sugar, causing it to spike rapidly. It's classified as having a high glycemic index. Brown rice, in contrast, is digested more slowly, causing a lower and more gentle change in blood sugar. It has a low glycemic index.

Diets filled with high-glycemic-index foods, which cause quick and strong increases in blood sugar levels, have been linked to an increased risk for both diabetes and heart disease. On the other hand, lower GI foods have been shown to help control type 2 diabetes.

One of the most important factors that determine a food's glycemic index is how highly processed its carbohydrates are. Processing carbohydrates removes the fiber-rich outer bran and the vitamin- and mineral-rich inner germ, leaving mostly the starchy endosperm.

Other factors that influence how quickly the carbohydrates in food raise blood sugar include:

- ***Fiber content.*** Fiber shields the starchy carbohydrates in food immediate and rapid attack by digestive enzymes. This slows the release of sugar molecules into the bloodstream.
- ***Ripeness.*** Ripe fruits and vegetables tend to have more sugar than unripe ones, and so tend to have a higher glycemic index.
- ***Type of starch.*** Starch comes in many different configurations. Some are easier to break into sugar molecules than others. The starch in potatoes, for example, is digested and absorbed into the blood stream relatively quickly.
- ***Fat content and acid content.*** The more fat or acid a food contains, the slower its carbohydrates are converted to sugar and absorbed into the blood stream.
- ***Physical form.*** Finely ground grain is more rapidly digested, and so has a higher glycemic index, than more coarsely ground grain.

All these elements lead to sometimes counterintuitive results. Some foods that contain complex carbohydrates, such as potatoes, quickly raise blood sugar levels, while some foods that contain simple carbohydrates, such as whole fruit, raise blood sugar levels more slowly.

There is one thing that a food's glycemic index does not tell us: the relative amount of carbohydrate in a given food. Take watermelon as an example; the sweet-tasting fruit has a high glycemic index. But a slice of watermelon has only a small amount of carbohydrate per serving (as the name suggests, watermelon is made up mostly of water). Looking at the glycemic index alone may not tell us everything we need to know about a food's impact on blood sugar levels. So researchers have developed a new way of classifying foods that takes into account both the amount of carbohydrate in the food and the impact of that carbohydrate on blood sugar levels. This measure is called the glycemic load. A food's glycemic load is determined by multiplying its glycemic index by the amount of carbohydrate it contains.

Although the fine points of the glycemic index and glycemic load may seem complicated, the basic message is simple: *Whenever possible, replace highly processed grains, cereals, and sugars with minimally processed whole-grain products.* And only eat potatoes - once on the list of preferred complex carbohydrates - occasionally because of their high glycemic index and glycemic load.

Sugar Management

Digestible carbohydrates are broken down in the intestine into their simplest form, sugar, which then enters the blood. As blood sugar levels rise, special cells in the pancreas churn out more and more insulin, a hormone that signals cells to absorb blood sugar for energy or storage. As cells sponge up blood sugar, its levels in the bloodstream fall back to a preset minimum. So do insulin levels.

In some people, this cycle doesn't work properly. People with type 1 diabetes (once called insulin-dependent or juvenile diabetes) don't make enough insulin, so their cells can't absorb sugar. People with diabetes (once called non-insulin dependent or adult onset diabetes) usually start out with a different problem - their cells don't respond well to insulin's "open up for sugar" signal. This condition, known as insulin resistance, causes both blood sugar and insulin levels to stay high long after eating. Over time, the heavy demands made on the insulin-making cells wears them out, and insulin production slows, then stops.

Insulin resistance isn't just a blood sugar problem. It has also been linked with a variety of other problems, including high blood pressure, high levels of triglycerides, low HDL (good) cholesterol, heart disease, and possibly some cancers.

Genes, a sedentary lifestyle, being overweight, and eating a diet filled with foods that cause big spikes in blood sugar can all promote insulin resistance. Data from the Insulin Resistance Atherosclerosis Study suggests that cutting back on refined grains and eating more whole grains in their place can improve insulin sensitivity.

No Carbohydrates

Some popular diets, particularly the Atkins diet, treat carbohydrates as if they are evil, the root of all body fat and excess weight. While there is some evidence that a low-carbohydrate diet may help people lose weight more quickly than a low-fat diet, no one knows the long-term effects of eating little or no carbohydrates. Equally worrisome is the inclusion of unhealthy fats in some of these diets.

If you want to go the lower carb route, try to include some fruits, vegetables, and whole-grain carbohydrates every day. They contain a host of vitamins, minerals, and other phytonutrients that are essential for good health and that you can't get out of a supplement bottle.

Adding Good Carbohydrates

Carbohydrates from fruits, vegetables, and grains should give you the bulk of your calories. For optimal health, get your grains intact from foods such as whole wheat bread, brown rice, whole-grain pasta, and other possibly unfamiliar grains like quinoa, whole oats, and bulgur. Not only will these foods help protect you against a range of chronic diseases, they can also please your palate and your eyes.

Until recently, you could only get whole-grain products in organic or non-traditional stores. Today they are popping up in more and more mainstream grocery stores. Here are some suggestions for adding more whole grains to your diet :

- ***Start the day with whole grains.*** If you're partial to hot cereals, try old-fashioned or steel-cut oats. If you're a cold cereal person, look for one that lists whole wheat, oats, barley, or other grain first on the ingredient list.
- ***Use whole-grain breads for lunch or snacks.*** Check the label to make sure that whole wheat or other whole grain is the first ingredient listed.
- ***Bag the potatoes.*** Instead, try brown rice or even "newer" grains like bulgur, wheat berries, millet, or hulled barley with your dinner.

- ***Pick up some whole wheat pasta.*** If the whole-grain products are too chewy for you, look for those that are made with half whole-wheat flour and half white flour.

Carbohydrates and the Glycemic Load
Low Glycemic Load

- High-fiber fruits and vegetables (not including potatoes)
- Bran cereals (1 oz)
- Many legumes, including chick peas, kidney beans, black beans, lentils, pinto beans (5 oz cooked, approx. 3/4 cup

Medium Glycemic Load

- Pearled barley : 1 cup cooked
- Brown rice : 3/4 cup cooked
- Oatmeal : 1 cup cooked
- Bulgur : 3/4 cup cooked
- Rice cakes : 3 cakes
- Whole grain breads : 1 slice
- Whole-grain pasta : 1¼ cup cooked
- No-sugar added fruit juices : 8 oz

High Glycemic Load

- Baked potato
- French fries
- Refined cereal products : 1 oz
- Sugar-sweetened beverages : 12 oz
- Jelly beans : 10 large or 30 small
- Candy bars : 1 2-oz bar or 3 mini bars
- Couscous : 1 cup cooked
- Cranberry juice cocktail : 8 oz
- White basmati rice : 1 cup cooked
- White-flour pasta : 1¼ cup cooked

[illegible]

- [illegible] whole grain [illegible]

[illegible]

[illegible] including potatoes

[illegible]

Baked beans

Fresh fruit

- [illegible]
- Jelly beans: 10 large or 40 small
- [illegible] bars
- Couscous: 1 cup cooked
- [illegible] juice cocktail: 8 oz
- White basmati rice: 1 cup cooked
- White [illegible] rice: 1 cup cooked

6
Energy

To understand this, you will need to remember a basic principle (of thermodynamics) that you have learned somewhere before in your educational career : *energy cannot be created or destroyed, but it can be converted from one form into another*. Energy has many forms... one form is chemical energy, which is the type stored within chemical bonds in molecules like glucose and ATP. Another type of energy is heat. You have already seen, back in the muscle chapter, that when we use lots of ATP in our muscles, like during a long workout, some of the energy from the ATP is lost as heat, and so our muscles heat up. That is an example of energy changing forms. Therefore, energy can be measured as chemical energy or heat energy, or even other types of energy. But the easiest measurement to make is in terms of heat - all you need is a thermometer! So, energy is typically measured in heat units called *calories*.

Calories relate back to the temperature you would measure with a thermometer in the following way. If 1000 calories of heat are released in water, the temperature of the water would increase by 1 °C. Water is specified, because different materials accept heat (conduct heat) differently. Nutritionists need to be able to talk about a lot of calories, so it is more useful for nutritionists to talk about *kilocalories* (which are also called *Calories* with a capital "C," or "large calories"). A kilocalorie, abbreviated *kcal* or just *Cal*, is the amount of heat required to raise the temperature of water 1°C, and is equal to 1000 calories.

One can relate the amount of each organic molecule consumed back to its caloric equivalence. So, 1 gram of either carbohydrates or proteins yields 4.1 calories of energy. And 1 gram of fats ingested yields 9.5 calories (more than double the amount carbohydrates and proteins yield).

Energy Needs

The amount of energy that we need can be described by our rate of energy consumption. Let's consider our rate of energy consumption at times when we are resting. This rate is called the *basal metabolic rate*, or *BMR*. If you think about it, the amount of energy that we consume should be proportional to the amount of energy that we make. And the amount of energy that we make stems from our rate of cellular respiration. The rate of cellular respiration is mainly dependent on our aerobic respiration, which requires oxygen (and glucose or its breakdown products) to occur. Therefore, BMR is proportional to the rate of our oxygen consumption. So, one's BMR can be evaluated somewhat by one's rate and volume of breathing at rest.

On average, a person's BMR is one kcal/hr for each kilogram (kg) of body weight. Since 1 kg = 2.7 lb, a person with a body weight of 150 lb can also be described as having a body weight of 55.6 kg. This person would then use *at least* 55.6 kcal every hour of every day. Over 24 hours this person would use 1362 kcal. This number of 1362 kcal would require that our average person be lying down and not doing anything for all 24 hours. Even just sitting up would increase energy consumption. Your book has a table, Table 18.4, where they show you how many more calories (NOT kcal, even though they capitalize it!) per hour a person would consume by various activities. For example, just walking around at a slow, meandering pace consumes 200 extra calories per hour, or (200 cal * 12 hr =) 2400 cal, or 2.4 kcal extra if you walk around for half the day.

Your energy needs are equal to the amount of energy you will be using in the day. You need to consume a little more than just your energy needs in order to replenish your essential-nutrients-stock. However, to maintain your weight, you should not eat much more than what you will use in a day. For example, if you eat an additional 3500 calories in a day, over the amount you will use, you will gain one pound!

7
Lipid

While too much fat is bad for your health, we do need some to survive. By cutting down on your fat intake you can reduce your chances of developing heart disease or cancer, not to mention staying in better physical shape and maintaining a healthy weight. There are three types of fat: saturated, monounsaturated and polyunsaturated. Saturated fats are the worst type because they raise the cholesterol level in your blood, which can lead to heart disease. The more saturated the fat is, the more solid it will appear at room temperature. This includes animal products such as butter, cheese, milk and meats. Monounsaturated fats are the types in nuts and fruit and polyunsaturated fats are found in oils. If you are trying to reduce the fat content in your diet, try broiling rather than frying your food, use skim milk rather than whole milk, use low-fat salad dressing or yogurt, and cut down on red meats.

Lipids are fats. Remember, lipids are not made out of building blocks like carbohydrates, proteins, and nucleic acids. Instead, there are just different types of lipids. Here are the types of lipids that you have learned about :

triglycerides (oils and lard)

phospholipids (membrane lipids)

steroids (cholesterol and hormones)

The main thing that these types of lipids have in common is that they are all insoluble in water. Also, triglycerides and phospholipids both contain fatty acids and glycerol.

Role of Lipids

As far as quantity of a type of lipid, we mainly ingest triglycerides. We get them whenever we eat butter, oil, or animal fat. Of course, we also get phospholipids and steroids (mainly cholesterol) in our diets, just not as much as the triglycerides. A few phospholipids that we need are ones with fatty acids that we cannot make from scratch— therefore, we have to ingest certain fatty acids. The fatty acids that we have to ingest are called essential fatty acids (and we get them in our normal diets).

Triglycerides are mainly used for energy or energy reserves. You see, we can break down triglycerides and use the products of this breakdown for cellular respiration, or we can store triglycerides as fat. This requires a bit more of an explanation. After we eat triglycerides, our digestive system breaks them down into fatty acids and glycerol for absorption. This absorption is shown a bit in Figure 17.44 (on page 690). The fatty acids are absorbed for the production of chylomicrons. Fatty acids enter the epithelial cells of the small intestine and are turned into chylomicrons with the help of the smooth endoplasmic reticulum. Once the chylomicrons are formed, they diffuse into the lacteal and eventually find their way back into the blood. Fatty acids can be drawn out of the chylomicrons into tissues that need them as the chylomicrons travel through the blood.

Fatty acids can be used in cellular respiration— they do not have to be turned into glucose first. Instead, the fatty acids are broken down into 2-carbon molecules that enter the cellular respiration events to make ATP. You see, glucose, a 6-carbon molecule, gets broken down into 3-carbon and then 2-carbon molecules as it goes through cellular respiration. Therefore, the 2-carbon molecules from fatty acids just join into the process where the 2-carbon molecules are normally used. Because they join in a little late in the process, they don't yield as much energy as glucose does, but they still generate some ATP.

Fatty acids can also be used to build storage triglycerides (fat for later use) and phospholipids for our membranes.

Cholesterol is important for manufacturing certain hormones, for helping to make up the lipid bilayer of cells, and for making bile salts.

Micronutrients of Lipid

There really isn't such a thing. Fatty acids and steroids are about as small as they get.

Storing lipids

In the carbohydrate page I gave you names for the chemical reactions that occur to make or breakdown carbohydrates. Here, there are no analogous names that you need to know. But, I would like you to know that the liver orchestrates the breakdown and synthesis of lipids.

Need of lipids

We don't need much lipid— only enough to get the essential fatty acids. Other than that, we can always make what we need. It is recommended that a person eat less than 30% of their daily calories from lipids

There are three main ways the body uses fats :

- Structural - Our bodies need fat as a building block. It is incorporated into cell membranes and other body structures, and used in fatty tissue.
- Metabolic - Affects hormones, including prostaglandins which affect metabolism.
- As fuel - It can be burned for energy. In fact, it is the body's preferred source of energy.

As well as that, fats are a valuable source of micronutrients, some of which can't be obtained from other foods.

So it is very important to eat enough fat, but also to make sure we eat the right kinds of fats. The wrong ones can have a profound effect on many body functions. There are two main debates about fat - how much you should eat, and which kinds you should eat. Let's look first at the different types of fat.

Types of Fat

There are several different ways of defining fats :

- Degree of saturation - saturated, monounsaturated and polyunsaturated. This is the main way that people differentiate fats and we'll go into that in more depth shortly.
- Animal fats vs. vegetable oils. This largely ties in with degree of saturation, with animal fats and tropical oils being mostly saturated, and vegetable oils being mostly unsaturated.
- Chain length. Short and medium chain fatty acids are found in butterfat and tropical oils, have anti-microbial & immune enhancing properties and are easily absorbed for energy, making them less likely to cause weight gain. This is why MCT (or Medium Chain Triglycerides) are often used in sports supplements. Unsaturated fats are generally made up of long or very long chain fatty acids.
- Cist form vs. Trans form. In nature, most fats occur in a "cist" form. In this form, they "fit" the fat receptors in your body, and can be utilized. Modern processing methods (including heating, hydrogenation, bleaching and deodorizing) turn cist fats into trans fats, which no longer fit. Your body still tries to use them, but they don't do the job properly and disrupt your cellular metabolism, resulting in a variety of health hazards.

Saturated Fats

Saturated fats are straight chains of carbon and hydrogen that pack together easily so that they are relatively solid at room temperature. They are found predominantly in animal products and tropical oils.

Monounsaturated Fats

Monounsaturated fats have one double carbon bond, which means they are missing two hydrogen atoms. They are usually liquid at room temperature, but solidify when refrigerated. They are quite stable. They are mostly found in olives, nuts and avocados.

Polyunsaturated Fats

Polyunsaturated fatty acids come mostly from oils extracted from seeds. Their molecules have kinks in them at the point of the unsaturated double bonds. They do not pack together easily and therefore tend to be liquid at room temperature. These oils are extremely unstable and go rancid very easily.

Fats and Cholesterol : Good, Bad, and Healthy Diet

"Eat a low-fat, low-cholesterol diet." Most of us have heard this simple recommendation so often over the past two decades that we can recite it in our sleep. Touted as a way to lose weight and prevent cancer and heart disease, it's no wonder much of the nation - and food producers - hopped on board.

Unfortunately, this simple message is now largely out of date. Detailed research -much of it done at Harvard - shows that the total amount of fat in the diet, whether high or low, isn't really linked with disease. What really matters is the type of fat in the diet.Bad fats increase the risk for certain diseases and good fats lower the risk. The key is to substitute good fats for bad fats.

Although it is still important to limit the amount of cholesterol your eat, especially if you have diabetes, dietary cholesterol isn't nearly the villain it's been portrayed to be. Cholesterol in the bloodstream is what's most important. High blood cholesterol levels greatly increase the risk for heart disease. But the average person makes about 75% of blood cholesterol in his or her liver, while only about 25% is absorbed from food. The biggest influence on blood cholesterol level is the mix of fats in the diet.

Dietary Fats

Type of Fat	*Main Source*	*State at Room Temperature*	*Effect on Cholesterol Levels*
Monounsaturated	Olives; olive oil, canola oil, peanut oil; cashews, almonds, peanuts, and most other nuts; avocados	Liquid	Lowers LDL; raises HDL
Polyunsaturated	Corn, soybean, safflower, and cotton seed oils; fish	Liquid	Lowers LDL; raises HDL
Saturated	Whole milk, butter, cheese, and ice cream; red meat; chocolate; coconuts, coconut milk, and coconut oil	Solid	Raises both LDL and HDL
Trans	Most margarines; vegetable shortening; partially hydrogenated vegetable oil; deep - fried chips; many fast foods; most commercial baked goods	Solid or semi-solid	Raises LDL

The Bad Fats

Some fats are bad because they tend to worsen blood cholesterol levels.

Saturated Fats

Saturated fats are mainly animal fats. They are found in meat, seafood, whole-milk dairy products (cheese, milk, and ice cream), poultry skin, and egg yolks. Some plant foods are also high in saturated fats, including coconut and coconut oil, palm oil, and palm kernel oil. Saturated fats raise total blood cholesterol levels more than dietary cholesterol because they tend to boost both good HDL and bad LDL cholesterol. The net effect is negative, meaning it's important to limit saturated fats.

Trans Fats

Trans fatty acids are fats produced by heating liquid vegetable oils in the presence of hydrogen. This process is known as hydrogenation. The more hydrogenated an oil is, the harder it will be at room temperature. For example, a spreadable tub margarine is less hydrogenated and so has fewer trans fats than a stick margarine.

Most of the trans fats in the American diet are found in commercially prepared baked goods, margarines, snack foods, and processed foods. Commercially prepared fried foods, like French fries and onion rings, also contain a good deal of trans fat.

Trans fats are even worse for cholesterol levels than saturated fats because they raise bad LDL and lower good HDL. While you should limit your intake of saturated fats, it is important to eliminate trans fats from partially hydrogenated oils from your diet.

The Good Fats

Some fats are good because they can improve blood cholesterol levels.

Unsaturated Fats—Polyunsaturated and Monounsaturated

Unsaturated fats are found in products derived from plant sources, such as vegetable oils, nuts, and seeds. There are two main categories: polyunsaturated fats (which are found in high concentrations in sunflower, corn, and soybean oils) and monounsaturated fats (which are found in high concentrations in canola, peanut, and olive oils). In studies in which polyunsaturated and monounsaturated fats were eaten in place of carbohydrates, these good fats decreased LDL levels and increased HDL levels.

Percentage of Specific Types of Fats in Common Oils and Fats

Oils	*Saturated*	*Mono-unsaturated*	*Poly-unsatu rated*	*Trans*
Canola	7	58	29	0
Safflower	9	12	74	0
Sunflower	10	20	66	0
Corn	13	24	60	0
Olive	13	72	8	0
Soybean	16	44	37	0
Peanut	17	49	32	0
Palm	50	37	10	0
Coconut	87	6	2	0

Cooking Fats				
Shortening	22	29	29	18
Lard	39	44	11	1
Butter	60	26	5	5
Margarine/Spreads				
70% Soybean Oil, Stick	18	2	29	23
67% Corn and Soybean Oil Spread, Tub	16	27	44	11
48% Soybean Oil Spread, Tub	17	24	49	8
60% Sunflower, Soybean, and Canola Oil Spread, Tub	18	22	54	5

Fat : Obesity

It is a common belief that the more fat you eat, the more body fat you put on, and the more weight you gain. This belief has been bolstered by much of the nutrition advice given to people over the past decade, which has focused on lowering total fat intake while increasing carbohydrate intake. But it isn't completely true, and the advice has been misguided. For example, while Americans have gradually decreased the proportion of calories they get from fat over the last decade, rates of obesity have increased steeply.

Over the short term, following a low-fat diet does lead to weight loss. But so does following a high-fat, low-carbohydrate diet. Actually, almost any diet that helps you take in fewer calories works over the short term. In other words, low-fat diets appear to offer no apparent advantages over diets with fat levels close to the national average.

Although more research is needed, a prudent recommendation for losing weight or maintain a healthy weight is to be mindful of the amount of food you eat in relation to the amount of calories you burn in a day. Exercising regularly is especially beneficial.

Recommendations for Fat Intake

Although the different types of fat have a varied - and admittedly confusing - effect on health and disease, the basic message is simple: chuck out the bad fats and replace them with good fats. Try to limit saturated fats in your diet and eliminate trans fats and replace them with polyunsaturated and monounsaturated fats.

The trickiest of these to attack are the trans fats. That's because they lurk in many different types of foods and aren't always included on the food label. But as awareness about trans fats increases, more "trans-fat" free products are becoming available. Now there's even a trans fat-free Crisco! Labeling of trans fat content has long been up to the food maker's discretion. However, a report on trans fats from the Institute of Medicine concluding that there is no safe level of trans fats in the diet (13) has finally prompted the Food and Drug Administration to require that all Nutrition Facts food labels list trans fats by January 1, 2006. Some foods - mostly those that are trans-fat-free - already list trans fats. Until all foods do, it will take some detective work to determine if a food contains trans fats. Check the ingredient list for "hydrogenated oils." The higher up these are listed, the more trans fats the food contains.

Tips for Lowering Trans fat Intake :

- Choose liquid vegetable oils or a soft tub margarine that is contains little or no trans fats.
- Reduce intake of commercially prepared baked goods, snack foods, and processed foods, including fast foods. To be on the safe side, assume that all such produts contain trans fats unless they are labeled otherwise.
- When foods containing hydrogenated or partially hydrogenated oils can't be avoided, choose products that list the hydrogenated oils near the end of the ingredient list.

Margarine vs. Butter

For years, margarine was pushed as a heart healthy alternative to butter. Butter was known to be filled with cholesterol and saturated fat that were bad for blood cholesterol and increased the risk of heart disease.

Because margarine was made from unsaturated vegetable oils, it was assumed it would be better for the heart.

Unfortunately, research showed that this wasn't necessarily the case. Some forms of margarine - specifically the hard stick margarine - were actually worse for the heart than butter. This was because they contained large amounts of trans fats.

The Nurses' Health Study found that women who ate 4 teaspoons of stick margarine a day had a 50 percent greater risk of heart disease than women who ate margarine only rarely. So, what should you choose to use? The best option is to use liquid vegetable oils or a soft tub margarine that is labeled trans fat free or non-hydrogenated.

8
Vitamins and Minerals

These nutrients don't supply your body with energy because they don't have calories. However, they are necessary because they help your body convert food into energy. Using our car analogy, vitamins and minerals are like spark plugs in a car, not the gas. The thirteen vitamins: A, C, D, E, K and the eight B vitamins (thiamine, riboflavin, niacin, B_6, pantothenic acid, biotin, folacin, and B_{12}) can be divided into two types: fat-soluble and water-soluble. You do not need to consume the fat-soluble vitamins everyday in order to maintain their proper levels because they are stored in your body fat and liver. But, the water-soluble vitamins, the B-complex vitamins and C, dissolve in the water in your system. So, these vitamins should be consumed everyday (with the exception of B_{12}, which your liver stores).

Vitamin A	Promotes normal bone growth, healthy skin, hair and eyes, helps with night vision.
Vitamin C	Strengthens blood vessels, helps the immune system, heals wounds and helps heal broken bones.
Vitamin D	Helps absorb calcium for stro ng bones and teeth, your body produces this from sunlight.
Vitamin E	Ensures that Vitamins A and C are not destroyed by oxygen and are properly used by your body. Helps form red blood cells.
Vitamin K	Called the clotting -factor vitamin, it enables your liver to produce a blood -clotting factor to control and prevent internal bleeding.

Vitamin B-Complex (8 different vitamins and minerals)	Breaks down carbohydrates and fat to energy, works to give you a healthy nervous system and healthy skin, helps you digest food and utilize minerals in foods you eat, important in the production of red blood cells, and works with proteins to build and repair tissues.
Thiamine	Helps keep your nervous system healthy, breaks down (Vit. B_1) carbohydrates into energy.
Riboflavin	Breaks down carbs, proteins and fats so your body can use (Vit. B_2) them for energy and repair.
Niacin	Works with riboflavin to convert proteins into energy. (Vit B_3)
Calcium	Needed for healthy bone and teeth development, helps with muscle function, and helps blood to clot.
Iron	Ensures the body produces red blood cells -- which transport oxygen. (Needed to produce hemoglobin - the red oxygen carrying pigment in blood.)
Folic Acid	Needed to produce genetic material (DNA & RNA), needed during and before pregnancy to

Vitamin Classification

Fat soluble Vitamins	*Water soluble Vitamins*
Vitamin A	Vitamin B_1 (Thiamin)
Vitamin D	Vitamin B_2 (Riboflavin)
Vitamin E	Vitamin B_3 (Niacin)
Vitamin K	Vitamin B_5 (Pantothenic Ac id)
	Vitamin B_6 (Pyridoxine)
	Vitamin B_{12} (Cyanocobalamin)
	Folic Acid
	Inositol
	Choline
	Vitamin C

Mineral Classification

Minerals	*Minerals*
Calcium	Copper
Magnesium	Manganese
Potassium	Chromium
Phosphorus	Selenium
Sodium	Iodine
Chloride	Molybelenum
Iron	Boron

Zinc	Fluoride
	Silica
	Cobalt
	Nickel

Calcium

Calcium is needed for strong, healthy bones and teeth. Women, especially post-menopausal, are in danger of developing osteoporosis if their intake is not sufficient. It is also necessary for correct muscle and nerve action, it helps maintain blood acidity and assists in blood clotting, and maintains healthy skin.

Signs of calcium deficiency: Shrinkage of skeleton, osteoporosis, muscle cramps, tingling or trembling, eye cataracts, slow blood clotting, irregular heart beat, irritability, insomnia and mental disorders.

Copper

Copper is a trace mineral found in all body tissues. It helps the body absorb iron, helps regulate and stimulate the brain, helps protect and support the nervous and glandular systems, assists in forming muscle and bone, and assists in the pigmentation of hair and skin.

Signs of copper deficiency: Too little copper can cause fatigue, weak blood cells, impaired respiration, skin sores, and lack of hair and skin pigmentation. Copper deficiencies are fairly rare, but can be caused by mega doses of zinc or Vitamin C.

Types of Vitamins and Minerals

There are many types of vitamins. Some vitamins are water-soluble, while others are not. Some are needed to make other molecules in our cells (like vitamin A is needed to make the rhodopsin pigment in our retinas), others are needed to promote absorption of materials in our digestive system (like vitamin D facilitates calcium absorption), others can be used as coenzymes (interacting with enzymes to increase their functionality), and there are even more functions that we do not need to worry about in this course. Some our bodies can synthesize (like vitamin D if exposed to sunlight), and others we can only obtain by ingesting them (like vitamin C). If we must ingest them in our diets, as is more typical with vitamins, they are called *essential vitamins*.

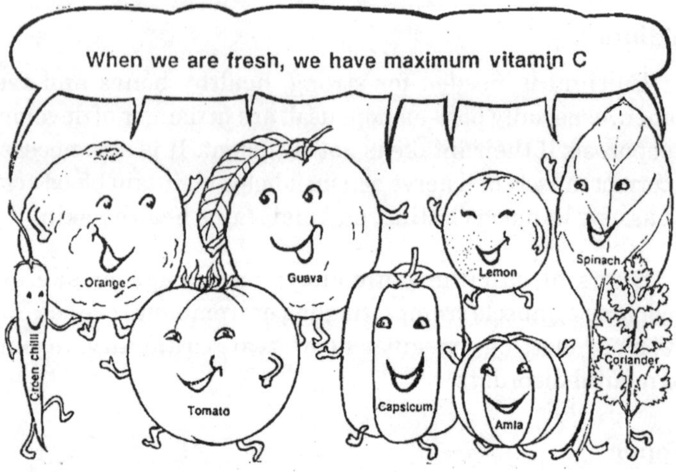
When we are fresh, we have maximum vitamin C
Orange
Guava
Lemon
Spinach
Green chilli
Tomato
Capsicum
Amla
Coriander

Vitamin C is fresh food Vitamins.

Minerals tend to be those elements that we need in small amounts, and we obtain them as atoms rather than in large

We help build bones and teeth.
CALCIUM
PHOSPHORUS
I am a component of thyroxine.
IODINE
We regulate fluid balance.
SODIUM
POTASSIUM
CHLORIDE
I am a component of haemoglobin.
IRON

Functions of Minerals.

molecules. For example, you know that iron atoms are needed in every hemoglobin molecule for it to work properly. Well, we lose some iron atoms every day and need to replace them in order to keep our hemoglobin working well.

Therefore, we must get iron in our diets. That is pretty simple if you eat meat, because meat contains some blood within it, and that blood has hemoglobin with iron in it. It is also pretty easy because if the meat you eat is liver, where iron is stored for recycling, you'll get tons of it. But, you can see, you have to eat the right foods to get the needed minerals. Or, you can take a vitamin and mineral pill to get them. Any way you go about it, though, you will need to ingest minerals.

9
Water

Nutrients

Nutrients are those elements from food and drink that perform a sustaining or metabolic function when taken inside our bodies. Essential nutrients must be supplied from an outside source because they cannot be made by the body in sufficient amounts. Water is an essential nutrient. Without it human life cannot survive. Water deprivation kills faster than lack of any other nutrient. If water is something you rarely think about, you are not alone. It is seldom considered a nutrient. Many people don't realize the important part water plays in major body functions.

Vital Link to Life

1. Water serves as the body's transportation system. It is the medium by which other nutrients and essential elements are distributed throughout the body. Without this transport of supplies the body factory would stop. Water also works as the transport for body waste removal.

2. Water is a lubricant. The presence of water in and around body tissues helps defend the body against shock. The brain, eyes and spinal cord are among the body's sensitive structures that depend on a protective water layer. Water is present in the mucous and salivary juices of our digestive systems. This is especially important for moving food through the digestive tract. Persons who experience reduced salivary output soon will realize that foods taste

differently and are harder to swallow. As a lubricant, water also is helpful for smooth movement of bone joints.

3. Water participates in the body's biochemical reactions. The digestion of protein and carbohydrates to usable and absorbable forms depends on water as part of the chemical reaction.

4. Water regulates body temperature. Our health and well-being are dependent on keeping body temperature within a very narrow range. The human body, which is made of 60-75 per cent water, serves this function quite well. Water itself changes temperature slowly and is able to help regulate body temperature by serving as a good heat storage material.

Evaporation of water from body surfaces also helps cool the body. Sweat loss that is barely noticeable occurs every day and night. Individuals may lose up to a pint of water each day in this manner. In hot, humid weather or during exercise, increased sweating and losses of water are more visible.

Water Balance

Each day water losses are balanced with water intake. The body has a sophisticated system that works to maintain water balance. Few of us ever experience malfunctioning of this system. Thirst is a trigger that reminds us to take in more water. At the same time our kidneys regulate urinary output.

Water : Daily Requirement

Unlike many of the nutrients, there isn't a specific daily recommendation for water intake. Part of the reason is the variability in individuals related to the climate in which you live, physical activity, age, state of health and body size. Under typical circumstances adults may replenish up to six or eight cups of fluid each day.

Typical water output is two quarts or more of water each day. Water losses in urine account for about three-fourths of daily losses. Remaining losses come from sweat, as tiny water droplets in the air we exhale, and through feces. Infrequent urination or dark yellow urine may be an indication you could use more fluid intake each day.

Water Sources

Water comes from a variety of sources. All beverages or fluids are a source of water. Even solid foods contain water. Lettuce, celery and other crisp vegetables are composed of 90 per cent or more water. Protein-rich foods such as meat, fish or chicken may contain as much as half to two-thirds their weight in water. Even grain products, which don't seem watery at all, may be up to one-third water.

Fats, such as butter or margarine, and sugar are among the foods that contain the least water. Some water, perhaps one to two cups per day, comes from inside our bodies as a by-product of energy metabolism. This amount is small but significant.

It is important to be aware of fluid intake. Even though solid food is a source of water, additional water from drinking fluids is needed. Besides plain water, juices, milk or other beverages boost fluid intake. You have a choice whether your fluid is simply water or an energy-rich beverage that may or may not contain other nutrients. Base this selection on your need for extra calories/and or additional nutrients.

Water : Special Needs

Under special circumstances, fluid intake and output should be more carefully monitored. Examples of the special circumstances follow :

Infants, young children and older folks : Children have lower sweating capacity than adults. They tolerate high temperature less efficiently. Frequent vomiting and severe diarrhea in infants and young children quickly can lead to water dehydration.

Older folks may be at increased risk for dehydration because their thirst mechanism may not be as efficient as at younger ages. The influence of medications and the presence of disease are other factors that affect fluid intake and water balance. For both the young and the old, encourage water intake often.

Athletes : Of all nutritional concerns for athletes, the most critical is adequate water intake. The athlete's immediate need for water is to control body temperature and to cool working muscles. Lack of water, above all other nutrients, has the ability to hinder performance and lead to serious complications. For example, fluid loss of 2 to 3 per cent of body weight by sweat- ing impairs performance. Fluid losses of 7 to 10 per cent of body weight result in heat stroke and death.

Two to 3 per cent fluid loss in a 150 pound individual represents three to four and a half pounds of body weight or one and a half to two quarts lost water. Marathon runners and other long distance athletes may lose up to three quarts (or six pounds) of sweat per hour.

To prevent dehydration during exercise, athletes should drink fluids before, during and after activity. Even exercise in cold weather results in sweat production and requires adequate fluid replacement. Although electrolytes such as sodium also are lost through perspiration, the immediate need is for water alone. In most circumstances sodium and other electrolytes can be replaced after exercise. Seasonings (especially salt) on foods at regular meals usually will do the trick.

During exercise or athletic events thirst is not always a reliable gauge of fluid needs. The best approach is to go into the event with adequate fluid intake.

Water balance in children involved in sports or physical activities is a special concern. Children have lower sweating capacity and less tolerance for hot temperatures. They need frequent fluid intake in order to regulate body temperatures. A water bottle or ready water supply should be handy during all sports activities.

Parents, coaches and others should remember that younger children also take longer than adults to adjust to warm weather following cool winter temperatures. It is especially important to watch fluid intakes during the adjustment time.

Outdoor workers : The combination of hot, humid temperature and physical activity places outdoor workers at special risk for water balance. Anyone who works or plays hard outside, especially in hot weather, needs to keep water handy.

Water : Other Elements

We often hear recommendations for increasing fiber intake in our daily diets. Adequate fiber intake is helpful for regulating bowel movements and, possibly, lowering serum cholesterol levels.

Persons with low fiber intakes who wish to increase their use of fiber-rich foods should increase fluids as they increase fiber. If not, they can experience extreme discomfort and risk having an impacted bowel. Dentists recommend fluoridated water for reduction of tooth decay. If community water is not naturally fluoridated, fluoride may be added. Fluoride concentration of one part per million (1 ppm) is considered safe while helping to increase the hardness of tooth and bone tissue. In some areas, natural waters are known to contain too much fluoride which can result in permanently discolored and mottled teeth.

Water purity in relation to nitrate content[1], bacterial contamination and other substances is a concern in some areas. Individuals who use private wells or water systems should have their water quality tested on a regular basis.

Water : Concept

Our bodies are about two-thirds water, and we need to ensure that we keep up this balance in order to remain healthy. That's why it is recommended that you drink at least eight glasses of water every day. This will keep all your organs hydrated so that they can function properly, and water also helps to flush toxins and other impurities out of your body. Water serves many other crucial functions including: respiration, digestion, metabolism, body temperature regulation and excretion. Water is also responsible for dissolving and transporting nutrients through the body. Only oxygen is more important to sustaining human life than water. So, drink a tall glass of water and stay healthy.

Water : for Life

Water is the very stuff of life and we need lots of it. Humans lose about 10 cups (about 2.4 liters) of fluid a day in sweat, urine, exhaled air and bowel movements. To replace that and keep a fluid balance, you need to drink between eight and 12 glasses of water a day, regardless of the weather. Caffeinated and alcoholic beverages don't count, since they are actually dehydrating and increase urine output.

Apart from those people who suck on a pump bottle all day long, it is likely that most people don't drink sufficient water. Fortunately, food makes up some of our water intake. A slice of bread, for instance, is 38 percent water and a medium baked potato with skin is 70 percent. In the average diet, solid foods provide between three and four cups of water daily.

Water : Function

It is generally accepted that water is needed to regulate body temperature, transport nutrients and other substances throughout the body, carry away waste and moisten, lubricate and cushion the body from injury. Since every function of the body is monitored and pegged by the efficient flow of water, "water distribution is the only way of making sure that not only an adequate amount of water, but its transported elements (hormones, chemical messengers and nutrients), first reach the more vital organs".

Water : Need

The need for water starts early, says Batman. "Morning sickness of the mother is a thirst signal of both the fetus and the mother." Batman argues that Alzheimer's disease is primarily caused by brain cell dehydration. In a dehydrated state many functions of the brain cells begin to get lost, such as the transport system that delivers neurotransmitters to the nerve endings.

Water, it seems, will not only enable you to retain your marbles, but also keep you spry. There is nothing better for rheumatoid arthritis than water, says Batman. Since the cartilage surfaces of bones in a joint contain much water, dehydration will have the effect of reducing lubrication in the joints and causing pain. Since 75 per cent of the weight of the upper body is supported by the water volume stored in the disc core of our vertebrae, sufficient water will also ease back pain.

But wait, there's more. Migraine, argues Batman, can also be prevented by regular intakes of water. Water shortage increases the potential for hypertension because the body copes with chronic dehydration by taking about eight percent water from blood volume. This causes some capillaries to close down, says Batman, causing hypertension. "Essential hypertension should be treated with an increase in water intake." Higher cholesterol levels also denote dehydration, since excess cholesterol is manufactured in the cell membrane to protect it against dehydration. "If you do not drink water before you eat a meal, the process of food digestion will take its toll on the body. Water will have to be poured on the food in the stomach for proteins to break down and separate into the basic composition of amino acids. In the intestine, more water will be required to process the food ingredients and send them to the liver."

Batman recommends taking one glass of water half an hour before breakfast, lunch and dinner and a similar amount two and a half hours after each meal. "This is the very minimum amount of water your body needs." Two more glasses should be taken before going to bed - water can also help you sleep. "Try drinking a glass of water and then putting a pinch of salt on your tongue. My personal experience and observation in others have shown that one begins to fall asleep after a few minutes. In my estimation, this combination alters the rate of electrical discharge in the brain and induces sleep."

When the body is well hydrated, one or two glasses of water "before the event" will help in achieving a firmer and sustained erection in men and joy of participation in women.

10
Planning of Meal

Introduction

The members of a family often have different food requirements. Their preferences as regards the foods also very. Some members have sweets while others prefer family tangy tasty favorites. Hence you may need large member of dishes a single meal to meet family food requirements. This situation is neither practical nor economical. Careful meal planning caters to most of the family needs, likes and dislikes.

What is Meal Planning

It is a technique of providing the family with meals that will meet their nutritional requirement. Meal planning is an Art as well a science. The meals served is an attractive way stimulate one's desire to eat. An individual salivates easily at the prefect of good taste. The digestive juices thus secreted go a long way in helping the body desire maximum food value. It is often called science because the knowledge of scientific principles of nutrition guide the home maker is making ins from the variety of foods available for optimum nutrition to all members of the family.

Hence, meal planning can be defined as the "implementation of the principles of nutrition in one's daily diet is an appetizing way".

The daily requirements of various foods are distributed over the day in different meals. In an urban family the meals are breakfast, Lunch, evening tea and dinner. This meal pattern is not rigid, hence, if can be varied to suit the and individual and family needs.

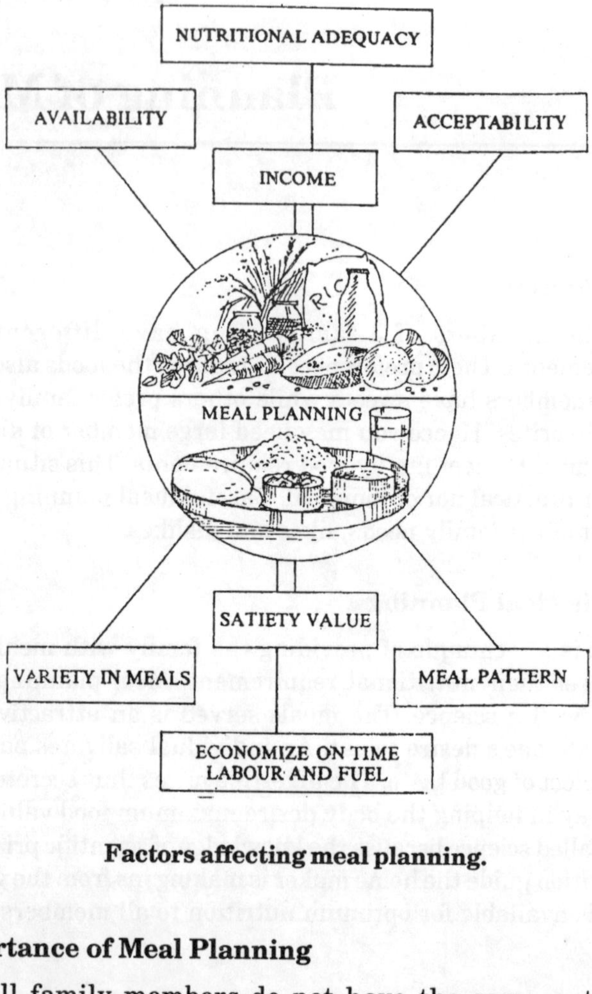

Factors affecting meal planning.

Importance of Meal Planning

All family members do not have the same nutrition requirements. Children eat less food than the adults. Grandfather may not be eating sweets because he is diabetic. Hence you ever seen a laborer eating his meal? He eats much more than your father. Hence meal planning is a very carefully drawn out plan of serving adequate meals to all the members of the family. The important factors of meal planning are as follows.

(a) Nutritional needs.

(b) Personal likes and dislikes.

(c) Serving Attractive meals.

(d) Planning Nutritional meals within the family budget.

(e) Good food combination.

(f) Using left over foods.

(g) Serving Time, Energy and fuel.

(A) **Nutritional Needs :** The protein requirement are high among growing children and hence they should be given sufficient amount of proteins of high biological value, e.g., milk, egg, and soybean etc. The protein requirements also increase during pregnancy and Lactation. After operations and individual should have high protein diet to promote to promote recovery. The calories requirements are high among active adolescent boys and girls. Athletes and laborers do strenuous exercise and work, thus require more of energy giving foods.

(B) **Personal likes and Dislike :** The meals planned for any individual should take into account his/her preferences. Children often dislike drinking milk which is an important source of most nutrients. Hence the milk can be given to them in the form of Kheer, custard or curd and the ice-cream that will be acceptable to the as far as possible there should be no compromise of nutritional needs on account of personal preferences.

(C) **Serving Attractive Meals :** I well planned meal should be appealing to the eyes. When you see an attractively served meat it creates an intense desire to eat it. It is rightly said that one eats with eyes finest. On the other hand what will your reaction be. If you are asked to take the sloppily served meal? Public eating places lay a lot of emphasis an garnishing and serving dishes to the customers. An intelligent mother and home maker will put in her best to provide attractive meals to her family. Her efforts will ensure good health for the family.

(D) **Planning Nutritional Meals within the family budget :** Food is expensive and hence a large chunk of one's income goes into the kitchen in order to provide balanced diet for all members of the family.

(a) milk, meat and meat products provide A- grade protein and these are expensive well informed housewife can use attractive foods to effect economy. Soya beans and Soya bean preparations can at times replace meat, Chicken, etc. to cut down the food cast.

(b) Seasonal foods are often cheaper than the off-seasons and convenience foods. Seasonal foods besides being tastier can affect economy. Seasonal foods are nutritionally superior to off-season and convenient foods.

(c) You get iron from green leafy vegetables. It is a common practice to discard radish leaves and eat the white root eating. Cook the green radish leaves, and you have a dish providing you iron at no additional cost.

(d) Lemons, orange and lime are expensive sources of vitamin E. Amla, Guava, and fresh salads provide all vitamin C. You need, but at relationally less cost. Experience and awareness as regards different foods will equip you to serve low cost but nourishing and healthy meals for your family.

(E) **Good Food Combination :** It enables one to plan balanced meals for the family. Rice is deficient in Lysine and pulses are deficient in methionine. The protein content thus improves if nice, and deal are taken together. Khichri, idle, dosa are some examples of good food combinations.

Deal are food sources of protein but when cooked in combination with green leafy vegetable improve considerably in iron content. Potatoes provide carbohydrates of combine well with a variety foods for making nutrition dishes. Can you name some of these dishes? Yes potato pea curry, Potato methi, Potato Palak bhujia, Potato Pakodas and Potato sprouted moong daal chaat etc.

(F) **Using left over foods :** It is important to incorporate left over foods to make a new dish. This way the monotony of eating the same foods, and the wastage can be avoided. Supposing your have left over deal, what can you make with it? Knead daal with atta, add coriander leaves, green chilies and chopped onion and make parathas with it. It sounds pretty in pressing to Pack with Paratha in your Tiffin box. Boiled rice can be used to kheer, and Lemon Rice. Hence, the meal planning ensures prefer use of left over foods together with money saving.

(G) **Saving time, Energy and Fuel:** Planning of meals avoids unnecessary trips to the market to procure

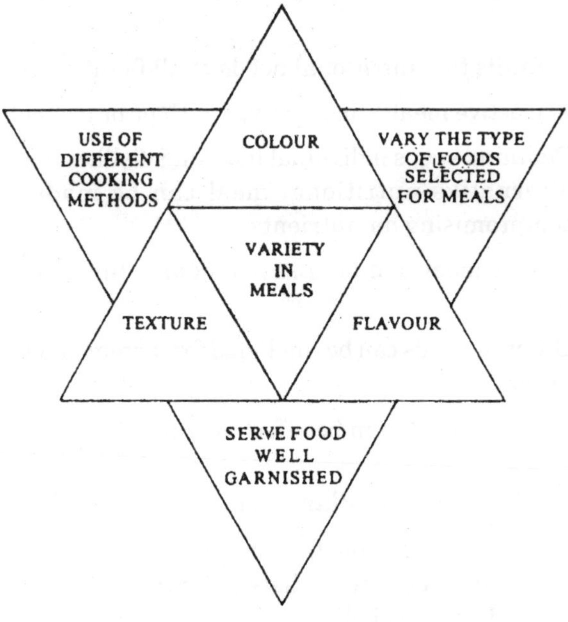

VARIETY HELPS TO ENSURE APPEALING AND SATISFYING MEALS

Variety of Meals

required food items. Planning of meals ensures organized shopping thus saving on both time and energy. Items required in large amounts also cast less when purchased in bulk.

It is desirable to use appropriate and simple methods of cooking to same fuel. You have studied the different methods of cooking in your previous class. This knowledge will enable you to cook foods for maximum nutritive value cook foods having simple recipes. Avoid lengthy cooking to conserve fuel. Make maximum use of pressure cooker. Use pressure cooker containers to cook more than one food at a time. It conserve a lot of fuel which is a lime resources.

Advantages of Meal Planning

The advantages of meal planning can be summed up as follows :

- It fulfils the nutritional needs of all family members.
- Attractive meals can be served with prior meal planning.
- Planning keeps individual likes and dislikes in mind and alternative nutritional meal can be made without compromising on nutrients.
- Proper meal planning saves money, time, energy and fuel.
- Different foods can be combined for increment of nutrient intake.
- Left over foods can be effectively used.

Factors Affecting Meal Planning

No two individual on families have exactly the same nutritional needs. Hence their diets differ in order to meet their physical, social and psychological needs. There are a member of factors which play an important role in meal planning.

(1) ***Adequacy of food.*** A good mean is one which will not only provide adequate accounts of fats, Calories, and

proteins but also minerals and vitamins essential for the physical well being of each members of the family. Therefore, the age, sex, occupation, physiological Condition and member of family members must be kept in mind. Hence for meals may very widely but an attempt must be made to provide a diet that will not lead to protein deficiency accompanied by a deficiency of iron. Sometimes deficiency of milk leads to a diet which is low in calcium. The of one on more foods from each of the different groups discussed will prevent most imbalances in diets.

(2) ***Meal Patterns must fulfill the family needs.*** While planning needs, one should candidate the needs and requirements of each individual member of the family. In a family there maybe a child, a man, adolescent boy & girl etc. Housewife who plans the meals has to see to their different nutritional requirements.

(3) ***Meal Planning should save time and energy and result in easy to cook meals.*** This point is particularly important for the families of low income groups or where the housewife is also working. If the meal consist of too many dishes and each takes a lot of time to prefer, then the housewife will spend for too meal time in the kitchen and become frustrated as other household chores remain complete.

(4) ***Individual likes and dislikes.*** Some people make personal likes and dislikes the only basis for the member on exclusion of certain foods in their meals – the failure to include milk is a common practice. It is always better to change the form of the food rather than to completely unit. For example – milk can be given in the form of curd, cheese, custard or another sweet dish, Soya beans in the forms of Soya for chapattis mixed with wheat flour.

(5) ***Suitable Combination.*** Food in suitable ways, variety in meals can be obtained and variety in meals means acceptability, thus ensuring better Nutrition. This can be introduced by changes in co lour, shape, texture, flavors and methods of preparation. Attractive combination, texture varieties, Flavors and methods of cooking play important role in it.

(6) ***Food should provide satisfy value.*** Food rich in protein and fasts have a higher satiety value compared to carbohydrates. While planning consider the interval between the two meals and accordingly include foods. If the interval is longer, give foods rich in proteins and fats. If the interval is short, then give carbohydrates foods.

(7) ***Availability of foods.*** The dietary habit depended mainly upon the foods produced a particular area or community, but today with improved methods of food preservation and distribution, even the mast perishable foods are available over large areas. The wide variation in dietary patterns throughout the world depends largely upon the available food supply.

(8) ***Economic considerations.*** The budget of a family of moderate means cannot provide luxury foods but it can definitely offer variety and choice. Food budgets of low income groups restrict the choices still function and it may become necessary to depend largely on cereals foods. The problem faced then is the supplementation of these cereals with foods necessary for a balanced diet. Although it becomes difficult to plan, it is nevertheless possible. When the cost per day is low, it is very important to have a good knowledge of less expensive foods which have high nutritive value. Such recipes and foods should be included in meal preparation e.g. paustik roti, seasonal vegetables, butter, milk, pickle or chutney.

(9) ***Seasonal foods.*** Today the seasons play a less important role in meal planning then in former times because fresh frozen foods are available throughout the year. Still foods included in the diet plans should be season because they are cheap and available in food quality and are within the reach within the reach of all people.

(10) ***Religion, Traditions and Customs.*** This is an important factor and food habits must be kept in mind while planning meals because they differ form religion to religion. Muslims can not eat pork, where as Hindus cannot eat beef. Rice is considered as an auspicious dish at festivals and marriage. Widows are generally not

served fish in Bengal. Customs and traditions differ from community to community and hence should be kept in view while planning meals for a family.

Occupations and Calorie Requirements

The approximate member of calories required per hour to perform different activities. These figures include the basal calories need.

Types of Activity	*Calorie/Hour*
(a) Sedentary activities Reading, writing, eating, Watching TV, sewing, Playing card, office sitting Work	80-100
(b) Cooking food, dusting, hand washing, articles washing, ironing, walking personal care, typing, office work	110-160
(c) Moderate activities Making bed, moping, sweeping Light gardening, walking fast, Setting office work	170-240
(d) Vigorous activities Heavy scrubbing and Waxing, Hand washing, Cloth washing, hanging Out clothes, Stripping beds, Other heavy work, golfing.	250-350
(e) Strenuous activities Swimming, Playing, Running, skipping, cycling, dancing.	350 and more

Flexibility in Meal Planning

It is very important to allow a certain amount of flexibility while planning a meal for your family. You have planned to serve mutton stew to your family and just then your vegetation grandmother arrives. What will you do? Cook special food separately for your grandmother on make vegetable stew instead of the mutton stew. However the later option is better for the entire family can enjoy the same meal with the visiting grandmother.

You had planned a rich, elaborate menu for the entire family. This food plan should be flexible in case of some family member falls sick. There should be flexibility in interchanging lunch and dinner meals on say Monday meals to Tuesday meal etc.

Guidelines for Good Eating Habits

(a) Maintain regular eating routine.

(b) Eat a whole lot of natural foods.

(c) Eat just right amounts foods, neither more nor less.

(d) Consume seasonal foods.

(e) Avoid excessive consumption of salt, spices, fats, sugars and sweets.

(f) Eat carbohydrates that supply plenty of fiber.

(g) Eat variety as it ensures supply of all essential nutrients.

(h) Maintain desirable height and health.

How to Plan a Meal for an Individual

Planning meal for an individual in a lot easier than planning the same for a family. Do you know why? Yes, you only have to take into consideration the requirements, likes and dislikes of only an individual.

Before you set out for planning meals refresh your knowledge about balanced diet and recommended dietary allowances (RDA). Given below is a sample menu for an adult women made for the recommended food allowances.

A Day's Sample Menu for an Adult Women

Name / Age		*Sudha / 30 years*
Structure	—	Medium
Activity	—	Moderate
Habit	—	Vegetarian

Food Allowances

Cereals	—	350 gm.
Pulses	—	70 gm.
Green Leaf vegetable	—	125 gm.
Other vegetable	—	75 gm.
Roots and Tubers	—	75 gm.
Fruits	—	30 gm.
Milk	—	200 ml.
Fat and Oil	—	35 gm.
Sugar and Jaggery	—	30 gm.

Recommended Dietary Allowances

Calories	—	2225
Proteins	—	50 gm.
Calcium	—	400 mg.
Iron	—	30 mg.
Vitamin A	—	2400 mg.

Meal	*Menu*	*Amount*	*Nutrient Provide*
BedTime	Tea	1 cup	Carbohydrate- Sugar
BreakFast	Paustik roti/ Parathas	-2	Protein carb.
	curd	½ K.	Protein
Lunch	Chapatti	3	Carb.
	Moong Daal	1 k	Protein
	Carrot & Methi veg.	½ K	Vit. A & Iron
	Papad	1	Protein
	Green Chutney	1-2 Tsp.	Iron & Vit.-C
	Radish & Tomato	½ Plate	Vit-C, Vit-A
Ev. Tea	Suji Upma	1 k	Carb.
	Tea/Coffee	1 cup	Carb-Sugar
Dinner	Steamed Rice	1 plate	Carb.
	Rajmah Curry	1 ½ K	Protein
	Chapatti	1-2	Carb
	Aloo Brinjal veg.	1 k	Carb-roughages
	Banana-Custard	1 K	Carb,Protein, and calcium

Note - You can plan meals for different family members following the pattern just studied.

11
Metabolism of Nutrients

The absorption of digested food is followed by assimilation. The assimilated food under goes chemical changes before it can be utilized to meet the needs of the body.

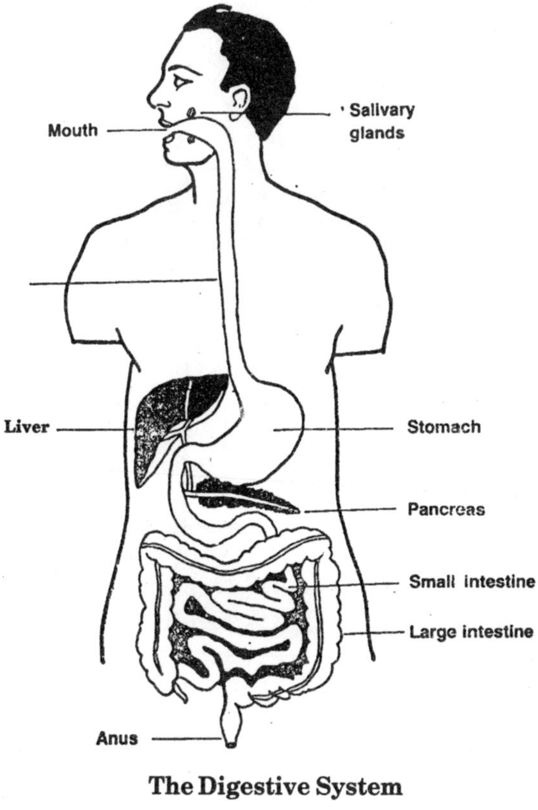

The Digestive System

Amino acids are used for the body protein synthesis in the body and also for maintaining and repairing of old worn out tissues. fatty acids and glycerol's provide energy to body and stored as fats in adipose tissues. simple sugars are used for energy and excess is converted into glycogen. Glycogen is used in the liver and muscles.

The break down and the synthesis activities that go on simultaneous in the body are collectively called metabolism. Meatbolism refers to all chemical reactions resulting in catabolic (break down) and anabolic (synthesis or constructive) activities. Catabolism refers to all chemical reactions of body materials. Anabolism can be defined as a process by which energy released due to catabolic activities is utilized for constructive and synthesis.

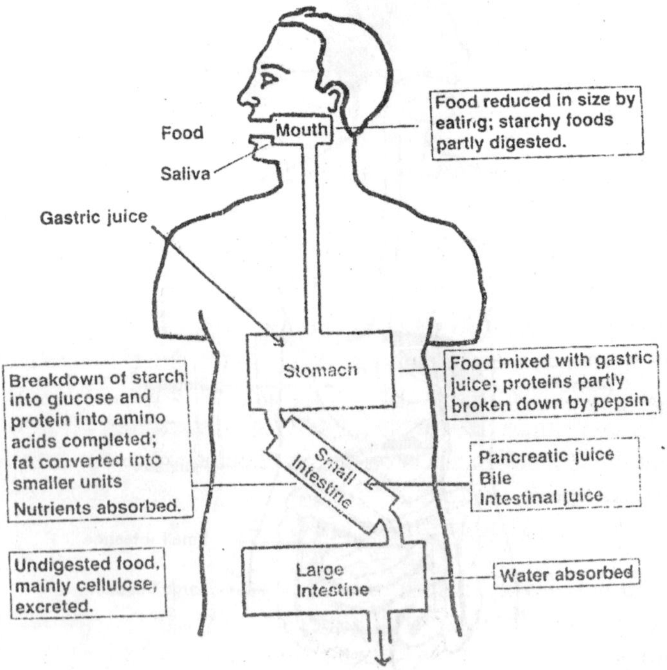

Digestive System

Energy Metabolism

Energy requires energy to carry on the voluntary and involuntary body functions. Energy requirement vary from person to person due to body temperature, environmental changes,types of food eaten, different psychological and emotional states also account for variations in energy requirements.energy is measured in terms of calories.

Calories requirement to raise the temperature of 1 gram of water. A physiological calorie is a thousand times more then the physics calorie. Food calorie known as kilocalorie.

Minimum calorie required to carry on the basic involuntary of body. The rate at which the calorie are required to carry on these functions in known as basal metabolic rate, of the individual and is commonly known as BMR. BMR can be commonly define as the energy expenditure of the body in a complete physical and mental rest. It can be defined as the rate at which a body is carrying on its overall cellular metabolism at basal condition.

Basal condition are defined as the past absorption state (12 hours to 15 hours after meal). Physically and mentally total rest in reclining position in bed in a room temperature of minimum 25 degree C in having comfortable humidity.

Energy out put and consumption of oxygen by living organism are dependent upon its muscular activity and other factors like the nature of food consumed,body temperature, emotional state of mind, age, sex variations. BMR can be measured by direct and indirect methods like spirometre readings.

Basal Metabolic Rate (BMR)

BMR rate depends upon the body surface and weight. In case of a 25 years old adult weighing 70 kgs. And having 1.8 sqms. surface area, the surface area per unit body weight will be 0.026 sqm/kg.

Children have larger surface area per unit body weight. This accounts for a higher BMR in the case of children.

The BMR decreases as children grow older. Hence age is one factors affecting the basic requirements of the calories. Boys are more stronger than the girls. The BMR of males is higher than the females. In cold climates the BMR rises, while in warm climate the BMR goes down. During starvation and malnutrition, there is a general decline in the body activity that account for a lower BMR the requirement of the energy increases when an individual is running a temperature. Every degree of rise in temperature calls for 12 % increase in BMR. Hormonal secretions affect the BMR of the individual. A person suffering from hyperthyroidism has a lower BMR and is slow and sluggish in his movements. An adults requires 1 calorie of energy per kilogram of body weight each hour to carry on with the basic involuntary functions. The BMR of an adult weighing 50 kgs. Will be $1 \times 24 \times 50 = 1200$ calories.

Calorie requirements as per body functions :

Light work	=	70 calories per hour.
Moderate work	=	100 calories per hour.
Heavy work	=	2000 calories per hour.
Very heavy work	=	300 calories per hour.

Metabolism of Carbohydrates

Carbohydrates may be utilized in the following process after digestion and absorption :

1. direct utilization.
2. temporarily stored as glycogen.
3. converted into fat.

The diagram indicates the direct utilization of carbohydrates.

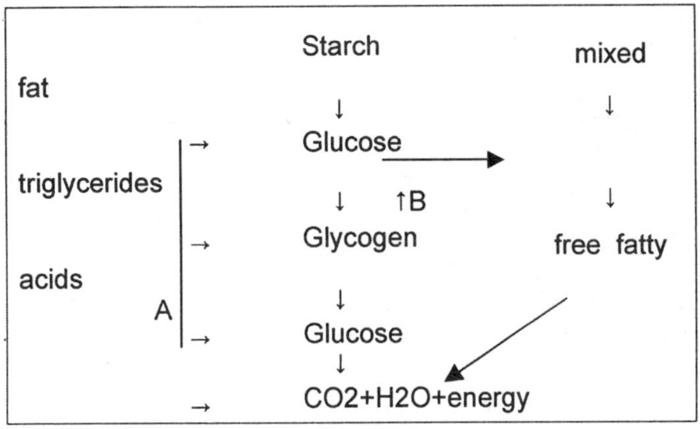

1. Direct utilization—glucose utilized by tissues of the body glucose is also called a prime fuel because it is the main source of instant energy. Small amount of glucose are found in the brain, but it is not used as a fuel because it maintain or remains fixed even when the blood sugar is so low as to cause neurological symptoms during starvation the brain maintains its glucose level even when blood glucose level is low. If the supply of sugar to the brain is cut off 9 over dose of insulin) mental confusion or hypo glycaemic coma will result.

2. Conversion into glycogen—animals, like plants are capable of synthesizing animal starch (glycogen or glucagons) liver has the highest percentage of glycogen. The glycogen in skeletal muscle is low but accounts for a large quantity of glycogen because of the large bulk of skeletal muscles. Glycogenesis is the process by which glucose carries by the portal system is converted into glycogen in the liver some of the glucose carried by the systemic circulation and is converted into glycogen in the tissues. The synthesis of glycogen from sources other than carbohydrates is known as gluconeogenesis. When the amount of oxygen in the blood is low as during excessive exercise more of lactate accumulated in the blood. This makes the muscles feel, taut and tender.

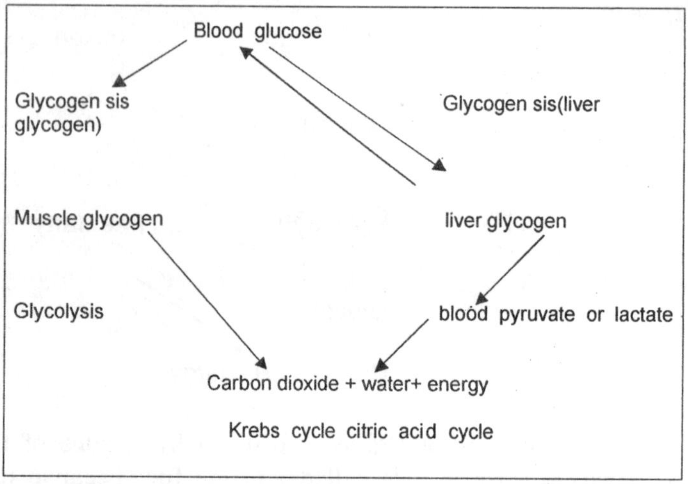

The diagram indicates the utilization of glucose in the body as below :

3. Conversion into fats—forty percent of glucose given to well fed animals is converted into fats and stored in the adipose tissues. The process of conversion of glucose into fats is known as lipogenesis. When ever glucose is in excess of the tissue requirements, it is converted into fat.

Energy requirement by the body can be obtained from the metabolism of fatty acids and the metabolism of glucose. After an intake of carbohydrates or a mixed diet, the release and utilization of fatty acids is reduced and oxidation of glucose takes place. The balance between fat and carbohydrates metabolism is brought about by certain hormonal secretions. These are :

1. Insulin—which is secreted by the beta cells of the Islets of langerhans in the pancreas.Insulin increases the the uptake of the glucose to muscles and tissues by increasing cell permeability and builds glucogen chain.The liver also stores glucogen.Insulin decreases glycogenelysis and increases glycogenesis with the help of key enzymes.Insulin decreases the blood sugar level.

2. Adrenaline—which is secreted by the adrenal medulla. Its effect is just opposite to insulin. It results in the rise of blood sugar as released from glucogen.
3. Glucagon—it is produced by the cell of Islets of langerhans. Its production is stimulated by hypoglycemia. Glucagon increases blood sugar due to break down of liver glycogen, which in the turn stimulated insulin secretion.
4. Growth hormone—it secreted by the interior pituitary gland. It increases the blood sugar level and antagonizes insulin action.

Regulation of Blood Sugar

The normal blood sugar levels is 100mg sugar/100ml blood.

The following diagram indicates the body maintains the normal blood sugar level.

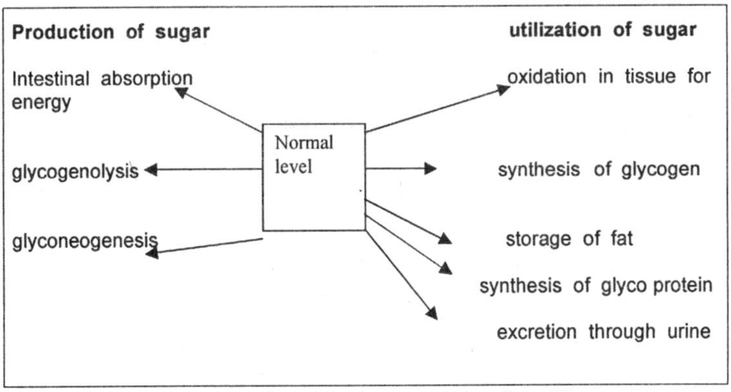

Diagram indicates regulation of blood sugar

The fasting blood sugar level is 70 mg/100 ml.

Post prandial state is -140 mg/100 ml.

Capacity of kidney is-180 mg/100 ml.

Glucose passes through the kidneys for filtration and its then renal threshold. When glucosuria condition the level is 180 mg/100 ml.

In hyper glycaemia condition the level is 100 mg /100 ml.

Carbohydrates has an action called protein sharing action when the liver can utilize protein to build its glycogen. The use of protein is wasteful and uneconomical as protein are expensive and more energy is used for the conversion of protein into glycogen the is liberated by the break down of glycogen itself. Hence a desirable diet practice is to spare proteins for other functions.

Metabolism of Fats

Fatty acids create as the breakdown of fats and glycerol during digestion and are absorbed in the intestine. Some of these used direct as energy and others may stored for future use,as long as chain of fatty acids which are stored in liver as adipose tissues.

In post absorptive stage - 560 mg lipid /100 ml blood.

The proportion of various lipids is as follows :

Phospholipids -	200 mg/100 ml. of blood.
Triglycerides -	150 mg./100 ml. of blood.
Cholesterol -	200 mg/100 ml of blood.
Free fatty acids -	10 mg./100 ml of blood.

Some lipo proteins are also absorbed by the blood soon after the meals. The plasma gets turbid and this stage called lipemia. The plasma turbid due to more lipids. Lipase breaks down as lipids thus bringing about the clearing of plasma called the clearing factors.

The liver play a vital role in metabolism of fat. Liver lipids form 5 per cent of the weight of the liver. When energy lacks the free fatty acids undergo oxidation and releasing energy. Under normal condition 0-40 per cent, triglycerides are taken up by the liver. Some fatty acids are activated in the intestinal wall and get converted into triglycerides.

Liver can also synthesize cholesterol and its esters. It helps in the production of hormones and bile salts. Regulation of cholesterol is done by the liver. In the body the cholesterol can be converted into 7 dehydrate-cholesterol which activated in the presence of sunlight to provide vitamin-D.

Triglycerides, phospholipids and cholesterol esters combine together and are covered with a thin layer of protein to form globules known as chylomacons. These gets absorbed in the systematic circulation. Free fatty acids form a loose complex with albumen and get transported to the liver and other tissuses. Sometimes the percentage of fat in the liver may go as high as 30 per cent of its total weight. This State is known as fatty liver. This condition may be due to over production of fat or decreased utilization or both.

In diabetes and starvation, the mobilization increased of fat from the adipose tissues resulting in fatty liver. Toxic substances like carbon-tetrachloride phosphorus and chloroform produce injury to liver cells causing fat deposition. Bacterial toxins can also injure the liver. Cholie, B_{12} and folic acids are known as lipo tropic factors. These help in converting phospholipids into lipo protein. Deficiency of these leads to impaired utilization and transport of fat from the liver.

The fuction of the liver is the production of acetone or ketone bodies. These are short chain products of fatty acids break down which produces energy to be utilized by the muscle. The process is known as Ketosis. There is 1 mg/ ketone body per 100 ml of blood. An increase form of ketone in body called ketonemia excessive secretion called ketoneuria.

Ketosis Condition

1. carbohydrate is low and fat level is high.
2. carbohydrate metabolism is disturbed.
3. fat metabolism is more.

The fat stored in the muscles and adipose tissue is not fixed or inert. It is in constant circulation. The fat deposit break down and mix with dietary fatty acids. This mixture is used for energy and the excess is again deposited as fat in the adipose tissues.

Metabolism of Protein

Protein play a vital role in the nutrition of an organism. they are necessary for carrying out a number of essential body functions.

The main elements of protein, breaks down into amino acids are absorped bulk the blood. A regular supply of essential amino acids, is required for the well being of the individual, while non essential amino acids can be obtained from:

1. dietary intake.
2. synthesis from amino acids present in tissues.
3. synthesis of amino acids from organic acids.

Amino acids are the building blocks for synthesis of cellular, sub cellular and other organic substances. All amino acids are joint together in different sequences and in varing numbers thereby giving rise to general thousand proteins tissuses vary in their chemical composition because of the presence of different amino acids. The brain is an organ that has a higher percentage of glutamine, glutamic acids and other non essential amino acids than other tissues.

Essential substances like lipo protein, albumin, glubbulin, and haemoglubin are synthesized from amino acids. Neucleo protein is conjugated protein and behaves as genes in the chromosomes. It is responsible for cell production, division and provides hereditary information. Hormones and enzymes synthesized from amino acids regulate body function and control the arte of biological reactions.

The tissue can hold only a small amount of free amion acids. Excess acids are diminished by the liver. The ammonia released by the liver is converted into urea and excreted as urine and energy utilized for the body mechanism. Amino acids can be converted into glucose that may be utilised or stored as known as gluconeogenesis. Those which can be converted to fatty acids are known as ketogenic amino acids. These give rise to acetoacctic acids and other ketone bodies. Deficiency and improper utilization of amino acids leads to serious consequences like low resistance, low plasma protein level and insufficient hormonal secretion. During this period the body is in negative nitrogen balance and draws upon " labile proteins" when the losses of nitrogen equal the intake,the body is said to be in nitrogen balance. During childhood, convalascene and pregnancy the losses are less than the intake and the body is said to be in positive nitrogen balance.

12
Food Preservation

Unless food is preserved in some manner, it begins to spoil soon after it is harvested or slaughtered. The main methods of food preservation that will keep food safe are canning, freezing and drying. Preserving food at home means having :

- An abundant supply of a variety of foods when the fresh products aren't readily available;
- Specialties such as strawberry-fig preserves or green tomato relish that can't always be purchased;
- The satisfaction of actually preserving foods yourself.

However, preserving food at home may not save you money, depending on the cost of buying or raising the food and the equipment, energy and time needed.

Canning

Canning is the process in which foods are placed in jars or cans and heated to a temperature that destroys microorganisms and inactivates enzymes. This heating and later cooling forms a vacuum seal. The vacuum seal prevents other microorganisms from recontaminations the food within the jar or can. High-acid foods such as fruits and tomatoes can be processed or "canned" in boiling water, while low-acid vegetables and meats must be processed in a pressure canner at 240°F (10 pounds pressure at sea level).

Pickling

It is another form of canning. Pickled products have an increased acidity that makes it difficult for most bacteria to grow.

Pickled products are also heated in jars at boiling temperatures to destroy any other microorganisms present and form a vacuum in the jar.

Jams and Jellies: have a very high sugar content. The sugar binds with the liquid present making it difficult for microorganisms to grow. To prevent surface contamination after the product is made and thus possible yeast or mold growth, jams and jellies are either canned, frozen or refrigerated.

Freezing

Freezing reduces the temperature of the food so that microorganisms cannot grow, yet some may still live. Enzyme activity is slowed down but not stopped during freezing.

Enzymes in Vegetables: These must be inactivated by blanching in order to prevent loss of color, flavor and nutrients. The vegetable is exposed to boiling water or steam for a specified time and then quickly cooled in ice water to prevent cooking. Blanching also helps to destroy microorganisms on the surface of the vegetable.

Enzymes in Fruits: These can cause browning and loss of vitamin C, and are controlled by the addition of ascorbic acid.

Drying

Drying removes most of the moisture from foods. Thus microorganisms cannot grow and enzyme action is slowed down. Dried foods should be stored in airtight containers to prevent moisture from dehydrating the products and allowing microbial growth.

Unsafe Canning Methods

Open-kettle Method : This outdated method of canning is now considered unsafe. In this method, foods were heated in a kettle, then poured into jars and a lid was placed on the jar. No processing was done. With this method there was often spoilage because bacteria, yeast and molds that contaminated the foods when the jars were filled were not killed by further processing.

The growth of these microorganisms, in addition to spoiling the food, often caused any lids that did seal to later come unsealed.

Steam Canning : This is a newer method of canning that is not considered safe at this time. The jars are heated by steam. However, safe processing times have not been developed and steam canners are NOT recommended for either high- or low-acid foods. Low-acid foods canned in these canners are potentially deadly because of possible botulism contamination. Also, both low- and high-acid foods are often very under processed and therefore could spoil.

Other Unsafe Methods : Canning food in the microwave oven, electric ovens, slow cookers or crock pots can be extremely dangerous, especially with low-acid foods, and is not recommended. So-called canning powders are useless as preservatives and do not replace the need for proper heat processing.

Adjustments for Altitudes

As altitude increases, water boils at lower temperatures. Because the lower temperatures are less effective for killing bacteria, the processing time must be increased for boiling water bath canning. For pressure canning, the pressure is increased.

The directions for canning foods are usually for an altitude of 0 to 1000 feet. If you are canning at an altitude over 1000 feet, check for altitude adjustments needed for canning each type of food.

On Guard Against Spoilage

Don't taste or use food that shows any kind of spoilage! Look closely at all jars before opening them. A bulging lid or leaking jar is a sign of spoilage. When you open the jar, look for other signs, such as spurting liquid and off-odors or mold.

Spoiled canned foods should be discarded in a place where they will not be eaten by humans or pets. Spoiled meats, seafood and low-acid vegetables, should be detoxified to destroy any poisons that might be present before they are discarded.

To detoxify canned low-acid foods that have been spoiled, carefully remove the lid from the jar. Place the jar(s) of food and the lids in a saucepot. (No need to remove the food from the jar-removing it could contaminate other items.) Add enough hot water to cover the jar(s). Boil for 30 minutes and then cool. Drain water and dispose of food and lids. The jars may be reused.

Improperly canned low-acid foods can contain without showing signs of spoilage. Low-acid foods are considered improperly canned and not safe if any of the following are true :

- the food was not processed in a pressure canner.
- the gauge of the canner was inaccurate.
- up-to-date researched processing times and pressures were not used for the size of the jar, style of pack and kind of food being processed.
- ingredients were added that were not in an approved recipe.
- proportions of ingredients were changed from the original approved recipe.
- the processing time and pressure were not correct for the altitude at which the food was canned.

Because improperly canned low-acid foods can contain botulinum toxin without showing signs of spoilage, they should also be detoxified and then discarded.

Surfaces that come in contact with spoiled or questionable food should be cleaned with a solution of 1 part chlorine bleach to 5 parts water. Wet the surface with this solution and let stand 5 minutes before rinsing.

Preserving Food at Home

It is possible to preserve food at home for people who are watching their salt or sugar intakes. Simply use methods that don't require sugar or salt for their preservative properties.

If preserving food for someone trying to cut sugar consumption, the food may be dried, or fruits may be canned or frozen in water or juice instead of a sugar syrup. The sugar specified in canning and freezing is only needed for its effects on flavor and texture. There are also many pickle recipes that call for little or no sugar. Sugar is the major means by which most jams, jellies and preserves are safely preserved. These products are not suitable for a person on a low-sugar diet. However, there are special low-methoxyl pectins and recipes designed to make jams and jellies with no added sugar.

It is also possible to preserve food at home for people who are watching their salt intake. The salt used in canning, freezing or drying foods is used only for its flavor or color protection quality. Pickling, especially when fermentation is involved, usually requires salt for preservative effect. Read the recipe. If it calls for a large quantity of salt, this can not be eliminated or replaced with a salt substitute. However, if the recipe calls for a large amount of vinegar and only a teaspoon or two of salt for flavor (not soaking), the salt can be left out.

Preserving Food

Vacuum Preservation

There are numerous types of equipment being marketed for vacuum packaging food at home. They vary greatly in technological sophistication and price, and usually are called vacuum packaging machines or vacuum sealers. These machines may extend the storage time of refrigerated foods, dried foods and frozen foods. *However, vacuum packaging is not a substitution for the heat processing of home canned foods.*

Vacuum packaging is also not a substitution for the refrigerator or freezer storage of foods that would otherwise require it. In fact, vacuum packaging can add to the concerns associated with storing of these perishable foods (which are foods not stable at room temperature and requiring cold storage).

There are many precautions that must be taken when vacuum packaging perishable foods for refrigerator or freezer storage. You must assume that the perishable food carries the risk of potential pathogenic contamination. And, when frozen food is ready to be thawed and used, steps to minimize the risks from microorganisms in food must still be followed. Again, perishable foods must still be refrigerated or frozen for storage after packing in a vacuum or partial vacuum environment.

Producing a vacuum means removing air from the contents of a package. Oxygen in environmental air does promote certain reactions in foods which cause deterioration of quality. For example, oxidative rancidity of fats in food and certain color changes are promoted by the presence of oxygen. Therefore, removal of oxygen from the environment will preserve certain quality characteristics and extend the food's shelf life based on quality.

However, removal of oxygen from the surrounding environment does not eliminate the possibility for all bacterial growth; it just changes the nature of what is likely to occur. In fact, what is most likely to be eliminated is growth of spoilage bacteria. The bacteria that normally spoil the quality of food in noticeable ways (odor, color, sliminess, etc.) like to have oxygen in the environment. If able to multiply on foods, these spoilage bacteria can let you know if a food is going bad before it reaches the point it makes someone sick. In an almost oxygen-free environment like vacuum packaging produces, the spoilage bacteria do not multiply very fast so the loss of food quality is slowed down.

Some pathogenic (illness-causing) bacteria, however, like low-oxygen environments and reproduce well in vacuum-packaged foods. In fact, without competition from spoilage bacteria, some pathogens reproduce even more rapidly than in their presence. These bacteria often do not produce noticeable changes in the food, either. In the vacuum-packaged environment, food may become unsafe from pathogenic bacterial growth with no indicators to warn the consumer; the bacteria that would also normally be multiplying and spoil food in ways to make it unappealing (odor, sliminess, etc.) are not able to function without enough oxygen.

For example, *C. botulinum* (a very dangerous pathogen that causes the deadly botulism poisoning under certain conditions) grows at room temperature in low-acid moist foods if the package presents anaerobic (lacking in oxygen) conditions – if the bacteria are present, of course. Without the competition from spoilage bacteria, reproduction is even easier. Refrigeration at 38-40°F becomes a critical step for storage of low-acid vacuum-packaged foods that aren't otherwise stable (don't keep) at room temperature (e.g., canned properly). The actual temperature of the refrigerator and the temperature at which it keeps the food are essential to maintain safety of this product. If the food were not packaged under vacuum, the oxygen in the environment would offer some protection against *C. botulinum* growth and toxin development in the package.

The removal or reduction of oxygen in the storage environment is indeed helpful for extending the storage quality of non-perishable dry foods such as dried nuts or crackers. Products like this are low enough in moisture that bacterial growth is prevented.

Vacuum packaging can also be safe for food that will be stored frozen. However, proper thawing under conditions that minimize bacterial growth – like refrigeration – would be essential. If the package stays closed during thawing, you still have a vacuum environment where pathogenic bacteria can be active if the temperature is warm enough.

There is no advantage to combining the use of a vacuum packaging machine with boiling water or pressure canning of foods. Jars processed in either canner develop sufficient vacuums for safe, stable storage at room temperature. They also have the added advantage of a heat process that kills pathogenic bacteria able to grow in that food at room temperature.

So is a vacuum packaging machine needed or are there advantages to owning one? One would need to ask if the amount of the investment is worth the uses for the appliance. Traditionally recommended freezing procedures and packaging methods, if carried out carefully, will produce high quality products with reasonably lengthy storage times. Storing crackers, nuts and other dried foods in air-tight storage containers will also keep them of high quality for a reasonable period of time for normal usage.

And, perishable foods still need to be treated carefully to prevent pathogens from making them unsafe. Remember, removing oxygen from a food's environment does not just solve some food storage problems – it could cause others. Consider how carefully safe food handling practices will be followed at all times, since vacuum packaging creates very good conditions for some pathogens to be a problem if any mistakes are made. For example, perishable food being vacuum packaged should not be out of refrigeration very long – no longer than 2 hours total time above 40°F. Food that needs to be refrigerated without vacuum packaging still needs to be refrigerated! While food is being packaged and prepared or used later, extremely clean hands, and clean and sanitized equipment and work surfaces are essential. Food should be dated and still used within reasonable storage times unless frozen. Raw meats, poultry and seafood should be cooked thoroughly to recommended temperatures, measured with a food thermometer, before eating. Any food showing signs of spoilage should be discarded – *when in doubt, throw it out!*

Food Preservation Methods

Research on food preservation is an ongoing process. The United States Department of Agriculture, the North Carolina Cooperative Extension Service along with many other groups continuously apply new research findings to their recommendations for food preservation techniques. The guidelines in these publications may be revised at any time additional knowledge is gained that may increase the margin of safety or improve the quality of home preserved products. However, the user must assume responsibility for his or her actions and use this information as only an additional source of information to help guide them.

Home Canning Fruits and Vegetables

To can means to heat process food in a glass jar with a lid in place. Heat processing kills microorganisms — bacteria, yeast, and mold — that contaminate food and cause food spoilage and/or food borne illness. Processing can be done in a water bath canner or a pressure canner, depending on the food's acidity.

High-acid foods (all fruits except figs that are not acidified) can be safely processed in a water bath canner. Acidified figs and tomatoes can also be safely processed in a water bath canner. Microorganisms in or on high-acid foods are easily killed at 212F (the temperature of boiling water).

Low-acid foods (vegetables and tomatoes that are not acidified) must be processed in a pressure canner. The bacteria that produces botulinum toxin cannot grow in high-acid foods but can grow in low-acid foods. The bacteria, *Clostridium botulinum*, have spores that survive for hours in boiling water. However, these spores are destroyed within a reasonable amount of time at 240F (the temperature reached inside a weighted gauge pressure canner at 10 pounds pressure and at 11 pounds pressure inside a dial-gauge canner).

If low-acid food is processed in a water bath canner, botulinum spores on the food will survive. In the absence of air, a condition found inside a jar after processing, the spores become living bacteria. As the bacteria grow, they form toxins. Eating even a drop of this potent toxin can be fatal to humans and animals. Many cases of botulism have been associated with eating low-acid foods that were improperly canned at home.

To make sure your home canned foods are safe, carefully follow the canning instructions in this fact sheet. Process high-acid foods in a water bath canner and low-acid foods in a pressure canner. Never process any foods in a conventional oven, microwave oven, steamer or dishwasher, as these methods do not kill microorganisms that cause food spoilage and/or foodborne illness.

Canning Equipment

Before each canning season, assemble and evaluate all of your canning equipment.

Canning jars— Use only standard canning jars (also called Mason jars) with the manufacturer's name printed on the side. These jars can withstand the temperature extremes of canning. And, the sealing edge is smooth and flat so lids will seal properly.

Never use commercial jars, such as mayonnaise and pickle jars, for home canning. These jars are not very resistant to temperature extremes; they break easily. Also, lids may not seal on these jars because their sealing edge may be rounded rather than flat. Finally, the neck of the jar may be so short that the screw band will not hold the lid firmly in place during processing.

Canning jars must be in perfect condition. Check all jars, new and used, for hairline cracks, chips or nicks on the sealing edge. Such defects can result in breakage or failure to seal.

Canning lids— The only safe way to seal a canning jar is with a two-piece canning lid. The set consists of a flat metal lid and a screw band. The lid has a sealing compound around the edge and is enameled on the under side to prevent food from reacting with the metal. The screw band holds the lid in place during processing. A vacuum seal forms during cooling, after the jar is removed from the canner. Screw bands that are in good condition may be reused, but always use new lids. Do not use screw bands that are bent or badly rusted.

Two types of canners— Use a water bath canner to process high-acid foods. A water bath canner is a large deep kettle that has a cover and a rack to hold jars. You can also use a big, covered pot that is deep enough to allow water to extend 1 to 2 inches over the tops of the jars with enough room for the water to boil briskly. Also add a rack to keep the jars off the bottom of the pot.

Use a pressure canner to process low-acid foods. A pressure canner is a deep, heavy kettle that has a rack on the bottom for jars to stand on, a tight-fitting lid with a gasket, and a pressure gauge. The gasket keeps steam from leaking out around the cover. If the gasket is worn, stretched, or hardened, replace it. There are two types of pressure measuring gauges, a dial gauge and a weighted gauge.

A dial gauge has a needle that moves along a numbered scale to indicate the pressure inside the canner. Each year check the dial gauge, old or new, for accuracy and during the canning season if heavily used. Call your county extension agent who has food safety responsibilities to find out where testing can be done.

A weighted gauge fits over the air vent tube. It permits pressure in the canner to rise to the desired point and then releases excess steam by "jiggling" or "rocking" to keep the pressure from going higher. Weighted gauges do not need testing for accuracy, but they do need to be kept clean. Check the vent tube to be sure it hasn't been bent or damaged during use.

Wash canning jars in a dishwasher or in hot soapy water and rinse well. Keep jars hot by leaving them in the dishwasher or in hot water until you are ready to fill them. Jars do not need to be sterilized, as this will be accomplished during processing. Jars must be sterilized if they are used for jellied products.

Wash and rinse screw bands. Follow the manufacturer's directions for preparing lids. They may need to be boiled in water for a few minutes before use.

Preparing for Processing

Fruits and Vegetables

Select high quality, unblemished fruits and vegetables for canning. Canning will not improve quality. Can them as soon as possible after harvesting. If you must store fruits and vegetables before canning, keep them in the refrigerator. If you buy fruits or vegetables to can, get them fresh from a local farmer's market, a roadside stand or a pick- your-own farm.

Thoroughly wash fruits and vegetables before canning even if they will be peeled. Garden soil contains bacteria.

NOTE : Potatoes must be peeled before canning. Potato skins contain a high bacteria count increasing the chance of botulinum toxin formation during storage.

Wash by scrubbing with a vegetable brush and rinsing thoroughly. Or, if more practical, soak in water for several minutes. Lift out of the water so the soil that has been washed off won't settle back on the food. Peel, pit, and/or slice only as much food as you can process at one time.

Some fruits and vegetables (apples, apricots, nectarines, peaches, pears and potatoes) darken when cut. To prevent darkening, keep raw, prepared produce in a solution of one teaspoon ascorbic acid to one gallon of cold water. Check among the canners' supplies in the supermarket to get this product.

Sugar and Salt

Sugar helps retain the color, shape, and texture of canned fruits. Sugar is usually added as a syrup. To make syrup, pour 4 cups of water into a saucepan and add :

2 cups of sugar to make 5 cups of light syrup *or*
3 cups of sugar to make 5 1/2 cups of medium syrup *or*
4 1/4 cups of sugar to make 6 1/2 cups of heavy syrup.

Heat until the sugar dissolves. Make 1 to 1-1/2 cups of syrup for each quart of fruit. Up to half the sugar used in making syrup can be replaced with light corn syrup or mild-flavored honey. Fruits also can be safely canned without sugar. Pack the fruit in extracted juice, in juice from another fruit (such as bottled apple juice, pineapple juice, or white grape juice) or in water.

Salt may be added to vegetables and tomatoes before canning. Because its only function is flavor, it can safely be omitted. Canning fruits and vegetables without adding sugar or salt does not affect processing times or microbiological safety.

Packing Instructions

The two methods of packing food into canning jars are raw pack and hot pack. Raw pack is packing raw, prepared food into clean, hot jars and then adding hot liquid. Fruits and most vegetables need to be packed tightly because they will shrink during processing. However, raw corn, lima beans, and peas should be packed loosely, as they will expand. For a hot pack, heat prepared food to boiling, or partially cook it. It should be loosely packed into clean, hot jars while it is still boiling hot. A hot pack takes more time but has been found to result in higher quality canned foods.

For either packing method, pack high-acid foods, including tomatoes and acidified figs, to within 1/2-inch of the top of the jar. Pack low-acid foods to within 1 inch of the top of the jar.

After food is packed into jars, wipe the jar rims clean. Put on the lid with the sealing compound next to the jar rim. Screw the band down firmly so that it is hand-tight. Do not use a jar wrench to tighten screw bands. There must be enough "give" for air to escape from the jars during processing. Process food promptly after packing into jars and adjusting lids. Processing times in recommended resources are given for pints and quarts. If you are using half-pint jars, use processing times for pints. For 1-1/2 pint jars, use processing times for quarts. Fruit juice is the only product that may be canned in a half-gallon jar.

Canning at Altitudes

If you live at an altitude of more than 1,000 feet, you will need to modify the processing time for high-acid foods and the pounds pressure you use to process low-acid foods. The processing instructions presented in most recommended resources are for altitudes of 0-1000 feet. After determining your altitude, your local extension center can help you to determine changes you need to make to your canning instructions.

Processing in a Water Bath Canner

Use a water bath canner to process acidified tomatoes, acidified figs, and all other fruits. There are no instructions for processing tomato products that are not acidified. A pressure canner can be used to process high-acid foods but the quality will not be as good.

1. Fill the canner half full with water; then cover and heat. For raw packed food, have the water hot but not boiling. For hot packed food, have the water boiling.
2. Using a jar lifter, place jars filled with food on the rack in the canner. If necessary, add boiling water to bring water 1 to 2 inches over the tops of the jars. Do not pour boiling water directly on jars. Cover.
3. When water comes to a rolling boil, start counting the processing time. Keep water at a boil for the entire

processing time. Add more boiling water to keep water 1 to 2 inches above jars.

4. As soon as the processing time is up, use a jar lifter to remove jars from canner. If liquid boiled out of the jars during processing, do not open them to add more. Do not retighten screw bands, even if they are noticeably loose.

Processing in a Pressure Canner

If you live at an altitude of 0-1000 feet and are using a weighted gauge pressure canner, process at 10 pounds pressure. If you live at altitudes above 1,000 feet, process at 15 pounds pressure.

If you live at an altitude of 0-2,000 feet and are using a dial gauge pressure canner, use 11 pounds pressure. If you live at an altitude more than 2,000 feet, you need to increase the pounds pressure at which you process foods. Contact your county extension center to get this information. If tomato products are acidified, they can be safely processed in a water bath canner or a pressure canner. Not instructions are available for processing tomatoes that are not acidified.

Here are some pointers for using a pressure canner :

5. Pour 2 or 3 inches of water in the bottom of the canner and heat to boiling.
6. Set jars on the rack in the canner. If you have two layers of jars in the canner, use a rack between them and stagger the second layer.
7. Fasten the canner cover securely so steam cannot escape except through the vent.
8. Once steam pours steadily from vent, let it escape for 10 minutes to drive all air from the canner. During processing, the canner must be filled with steam, not air, since it is steam that reaches the desired temperature of 240F.
9. Processing time :

(a) If the canner has a weighted gauge, start counting the processing time when it jiggles or rocks. The target pressure for this type of canner is 10 pounds pressure. Adjust heat so that gauge jiggles 2 or 3 times a minute or maintains a slow, steady, rocking motion.

(b) If the canner has a dial gauge, bring pressure up quickly to 8 pounds, then adjust the heat to maintain 11 pounds pressure. Start counting the processing times when the gauge registers 11 pounds pressure.

10. When the processing time is up, turn off the burner. (If you are using a coal or wood stove, remove the canner from heat.) Let the pressure in the canner drop to zero by itself. This may take 45 minutes in a 16-quart canner filled with jars and almost an hour in a 22-quart canner. If the vent is opened before the pressure drops to zero or if the cooling is rushed by cold running water over the canner, liquid will be lost from the jars.
11. When the pressure has dropped to zero, open the vent or remove the weighted gauge. (With a weighted gauge canner, pressure is completely reduced if no steam escapes when the gauge is nudged or tilted. If steam spurts out, pressure is not yet down).
12. Remove the canner cover carefully, tilting it away from your face so that the rising steam cannot burn your face or hands.
13. Remove jars from the canner. If liquid boiled out of jars during processing, do not open jars to add more liquid. Do not retighten screw bands, even if they are noticeably loose.
14. Place hot jars upright to cool on a towel or rack. Leave space between them so air can circulate. Keep jars our of drafts.

Check Seals

Vacuum seals form as the jars cool. When jars are cool (12 to 24 hours after processing), check the seals. If the lid is depressed or concave and will not move when pressed, it is sealed.

If sealed, carefully remove screw bands. If a band sticks, loosen it by covering, it for a moment with a hot, damp cloth. Bands left on jars during storage may rust, making later removal difficult.

If you find an unsealed jar, do one of the following :

- Refrigerate the food and use it within 2 to 3 days.
- Freeze the food. Drain vegetables before freezing.
- Reprocess the food. Remove lids, empty the contents in to a pan, heat to boiling, pack into clean, hot jars, and put on new lids. Process again for the full time.
- The eating quality of twice-processed food may be poor. If more than 24 hours has gone by since processing, throw out the food. It might be unsafe to eat.

Label and Store Sealed Jars

Label sealed jars with the processing date. Store them in a cool, dry, dark place. Properly stored canned foods will retain their quality for at least one year. Never store canned foods near hot pipes, a range, a furnace, or in direct sunlight because they lose quality.

If stored in a cold place, protect from freezing by wrapping the jars in newspaper or covering them with a blanket. Canned foods that do freeze may be used as long as freezing does not break the seal. However, they may not be as tasty as properly stored canned foods.

If canned foods are kept in a damp place, lids may rust.

Signs of Spoilage

Before using always check canned foods for signs of spoilage-leakage, bulging lids, or loss of seal. Bulging or loss of seal indicates gas formation inside the jar. After opening the jar, look for spurting liquid, cloudy liquid, disagreeable odor, or mold. Never taste food that shows any sign of spoilage. *Throw it out; it might be unsafe to eat. Furthermore, never feed this food to animals; it could make them sick.*

Cloudy liquid may be a sign of spoilage or be due to minerals in hard water or starch from overripe vegetables. If liquid is cloudy, check for other signs of spoilage. If there are no other signs of spoilage, boil the food. Do not eat any food that foams or has a disagreeable odor during heating.

Always boil home-canned, low-acid foods for 10 minutes before tasting. Do not use this method to make improperly processed food "safe." If enough bacteria is present (due to improper process), it is not certain that ten minutes will destroy the toxin. Black deposits on the underside of a lid are not a sign of spoilage. The underside of a canning lid is coated with enamel. If there are imperfections, such as tiny scratches or pinholes in the enamel, natural compounds in food can react with the metal in the lid to form harmless brown or black deposits.

Preserving Food - Drying

Drying is a method of food preservation that is simple, safe and easy to learn. Drying also creates new food products such as fruit leathers, banana chips, pumpkin seeds and beef jerky.

Drying removes the moisture from the food so bacteria, yeasts and molds cannot grow. Drying also slows down the action of enzymes, which cause food to ripen.

Because drying removes moisture, the food shrinks, and becomes lighter in weight. When the food is ready for use you add water and the food returns to its original shape.

Foods can be dried in an oven, or in a food dehydrator by using the right combination of warmth, low humidity and air current.

In drying, a warm temperature allows the moisture to evaporate. Air current speeds up drying by moving the surrounding moist air away from the food. Low humidity allows moisture to move from the food to the air.

Drying food is a slow process. It will take 6 or more hours in a dehydrator, and in your oven, it will take 8 or more hours. Drying time depends on type of food, thickness, and type of dryer. Don't be tempted to speed up the drying time by turning up the oven. You will cook the food on the outside before it dries on the inside. This is called case hardening.

The food may appear dry on the outside but may be wet on the inside. Moisture left in the food will cause it to mold.

After foods are dried, allow 30 minutes to one hour cooling time to prevent condensation. However, too long a cooling period allows moisture from the air to re-enter the food.

Proper storage prevents insects and rodents from eating food. It also keeps moisture out and saves valuable nutrients. Glass jars, metal cans or boxes with new tight fitting lids, or vapor-proof freezer cartons make good containers. The jars do not need to be heat processed. Heavy duty plastic bags with press together seals are acceptable, but are not insect and rodent proof.

Dried foods will keep from four to twelve months, but proper storage is very important. Cool, dry, dark are best. For best quality, the storage temperature should not go over 60 degrees. Refrigerator or freezer storage does provide a low temperature which extends the shelf life.

After packaging, check containers within seven to ten days to see if any moisture is present. If you see any moisture, food must be redried. If it is moldy, discard the food. Dried fruits can be eaten as nutritious snacks, or they can be soaked for one to two hours and used in favorite recipes.

Some vegetables can be eaten dried as tasty vegetable chips or used in dips. Most vegetables are refreshed with water before use.

Home Freezing of Cooked and Prepared Foods

Preparing food ahead of time and freezing it can save time, energy and money. Frozen cooked foods also add variety to your menu, offer quick meals for unexpected company and provide nutritious choices for busy days.

When you are preparing a main dish, it takes only a little more effort and time to make enough for several meals. You can freeze all of the prepared food in meal size packages, or serve part of the food immediately and freeze the rest.

It is more economical to make your own supply of prepared dishes than to purchase commercially prepared foods.

Consider freezing :

- Leftovers that cannot be used immediately.
- Foods that ordinarily take a long time to prepare.
- Seasonal fruits and vegetables.
- Foods you can prepare in quantity.
- Foods that still taste good after a reasonable storage time.

Hints for Freezing for long time

Select only fresh, high quality ingredients because freezing does not improve the quality of food.

Slightly undercook prepared foods. They will finish cooking when reheated.

Cool foods quickly before packaging. Place the pan of food in a large pan of ice water, crushed ice or cubes. Stirring will help cool the food faster. Use a fan to cool foods that cannot be stirred.

Freeze food promptly as soon as it is cooled to room temperature.

Put no more unfrozen food in the freezer than will freeze within 24 hours. Usually this is 2 or 3 pounds per cubic foot of freezer capacity. Stack the food after it is frozen.

Plan to use frozen prepared foods within a short time. Keep using foods from the freezer and replenish with fresh stock. This makes greater use of freezer space, lowers the cost per pound of food stores, and keeps your store of food fresh.

The temperature of the freezer should not go above 0°F. Fluctuating temperatures and temperatures that are not low enough cause loss of quality.

Foods that do not freeze well include mayonnaise, cream puddings and fillings, custard, gelatin salads, cheese, the whites of hard cooked eggs and uncooked egg yolks.

Hints for Packaging

Use freezer containers or wrappings of moisture/vapor-resistant material.

Pack food compactly into the container to reduce the amount of air in the package. Allow head room for expansion as food freezes.

In quart containers, the food may be separated into two or three layers by a double thickness of water resistant wrapping material.

Quart containers hold four to six servings; pints, two to three.

Choose containers by the number of servings you will want to serve.

Use only containers with wide top openings. Food can then be removed without thawing.

Freeze the prepared foods in your favorite casserole dish. The food can be removed after freezing, wrapped and returned to the freezer for storage.

For microwave reheating, use plastic wrap for wrapping small amounts of quick breads or breads. Casseroles should be approved for microwave use.

Label and date all packages, and keep an inventory of all frozen food.

Freezing Recommendations for Commonly Prepared Foods

Food	*Preparation*	*Serving*	*Storage Time*
COMBINATION DISHES	(Foods should be undercooked)		
Baked beans and other bean dishes Rice or spaghetti dishes Lasagna Chow mein Soups Stuffed peppers or eggplants Meat pies	After cooking, cool these dishes by setting pan or oven-freezer tempered baking dish in a shallow pan of water or crushed ice. Stir occasionally. Freeze promptly when cool. Wrap package compactly to eliminate air space. Meat pies need not be baked. Top crust may be sufficient.	Thaw and use only the serving portions you need. Reheat at medium temperature as appropriate --on top of the stove, use heavy sauce pan or double boiler; in oven at 350°F (400°F for meat pies).	2-4 months 3 months
MEAT, POULTRY, FISH			
Meat loaf Meat balls Meat sauce Veal birds Roasts Cubed or chunky meat Ham Turkey Chicken Fish	Prepare as usual, freeze raw or cook to rare stage before freezing. Meat balls can be cov ered with sauce. Do not stuff poultry. Remove ham bone after baking to save freezer space. Package in appropriate sized containers for later use.	Reheat in skillet or 350°F oven. No need to thaw. Cooking time will be 10 -20 minutes per pound.	1-3 months
POTATOES			
Mashed	Store leftovers in a straight sided container. Or add a beaten egg and shape into patties. Shape and store with double layer of paper between them.	Thaw just enough to slip potatoes into top of double boiler. Dip patties in flour and brown in fat at low heat.	2-4 weeks
Stuffed (baked)	Cut freshly baked potatoes in half lengthwise. Scoop out potato, leaving skin unbroken. Mash scooped out potato and season. Pile into shells. Cool and wrap.	Remove from package or wrap. Place on baking sheet. R eheat at 325-350°F until piping hot. Garnish; add cheese if desired.	1 month
French Fries	Use a high starch content potato for frying (Idaho or similar type). Fry in hot fat until a light brown.	Spread on cookie sheet and place in 400°F oven until thawed and crisp.	1-2 months

Sweet Potatoes	Dip boiled potatoes in lemon juice or package with cooking water around them. Freeze candied or mashed potatoes in a casserole. Leave skin on baked potatoes.	Reheat in 325 -350°F oven until hot throughout.	months
COMPARTMENT PLATES OR TRAYS			
• Roast beef, corn and spinach • Swiss steak, french fried potatoes • Sliced turkey, dressing or stuffed baked potato and mixed vegetables • Ham slice, sweet potato and broccoli	Food packaged together should be those which retain quality for about the same period of time, and require same heating time. Most vegetables need only blanching before freezing meat and vegetables. Sauces may be added!	Reheat with tray or plate covered, except for crispy foods which should be uncovered.	month
QUICK BREADS			
Biscuits Muffins Coffee cake Fruit bread Doughnuts Waffles Pancakes	Prepare as usual, cool. Freeze in pan and cover tightly. May be packaged in aluminum foil for reheating. Waffles and pancakes may be separated in layers in plastic containers.	Heat in pan or foil in 325-350°F oven until hot. Waffles and pancakes may be heated from frozen stage in the toaster until hot and crispy.	1-2 months
YEAST BREADS			
Rolls Sweet rolls Loaf of bread Coffee cake	Dough may be made, shaped, placed in pa ns and frozen; or baked before freezing. Cover uncooked bread tightly and freeze before product has raised. For baked bread, cool, then cover pan tightly or place product in foil.	For unbaked bread, uncover and let bread rise before baking. Bake at 350 -375°F. For baked bread, reheat in pan or foil at 300°F for 15-20 minutes.	3-6 months

SANDWICHES	Spread slices of bread with butter or margarine. Add filling and spread evenly. Wrap individually or in packages large enough to serve family. Thaw in wrapping.	Sandwiches for grilling, such as cheese or ham salad, should be thawed before grilling in frying pan, oven or on grill.	3-4 weeks
HORS D'OEUVRES	Small meatballs, chicken wings and pastry items. Can be made and frozen for future use. Use directions for freezing meats and pastries.	Thaw, bake in oven until done. Serve immediately.	2-4 weeks
CAKES			
Shortened (Baked)	Prepare and bake as usual in layers or loaf pan. Cool. Remove from pans and wrap tightly. Loaf cake may be cut to family size pieces before wrapping.	Thaw cake in wrapping at room temperature. Ice and serve.	2-4 months
(Unbaked)	Unbaked cakes take more time to thaw and bake than when starting from beginning. There is also a loss of volume. Therefore, use double acting baking powder in mixture and freeze in baking dish.	Thaw in refrigerator. Bake at 350 - 375°F. Cool. Ice.	2 weeks
Sponge cake, angel and chiffon	Bake thoroughly. Cool. May freeze before wrapping. Place in container that will prevent crushing. Wrap immediately after freezing.	Thaw unfrosted in the refrigerator.	4-6 months
ICINGS	Powdered sugar icings made with fat freeze well. Cooked candy-type frostings may stay soft and creamy between layers, but often crack and crumble on outside of cake.		
COOKIES			
(Baked)	Prepare and bake as stated in recipe. Cool thoroughly. Package in foil or rigid container. Place 2 layers of waxed paper between cookies.	Thaw in containers at room temperature. Remove from containers and serve.	6 months
(Unbaked)	Prepare your favorite cookie dough. Pour in baking pan, or wrap more firm cookie dough in foil or moisture/vapor-resistant material.	Thaw dough in refrigerator. Firm cookie dough may be sliced before completely thawed and baked.	2 weeks

PIES			
(Unbaked, 2-crust)	Prepare as usual. Pies may be frozen and then wrapped, or wrapped and frozen. Pies can be stacked after freezing.	Unwrap. Bake at 425°F for 45 to 50 minutes. Serve hot or cold.	2 months
Chiffon	Prepare as usual. Freeze, then wrap.	Unwrap; thaw in refrigerator from 1 to 2 hours.	1 month
(Baked, 2-crust) Custard Pumpkin	Bake until done. Cool quickly. May use fan. Wrap and freeze.	Unwrap; thaw in refrigerator and serve chilled or reheat in 375°F oven. Thaw custard and pumpkin pies in refrigerator or 325°F oven.	

Food Selection and Storage

Food quality and safety

Storage does not improve the quality of any food. The quality of a food will also not decrease significantly during storage as long as the food is stored properly and used within the recommended time frame.

Quality is not the same as safety. A poor-quality food may be safe such as stale cereal, overripe fruit or soured pasteurized milk. An unsafe food may have good quality in terms of appearance and taste, but have a high (unsafe) bacterial count. For example, improperly canned food may contain *Clostridium botulinum*) thus making food unsafe. Or cooked chicken may be placed on a plate that held the raw chicken and become contaminated. The goal of home food storage is to provide both safe and high-quality foods.

Maintaining a food's quality depends on several factors: the quality of the raw product, the procedures used during processing, the way the food is stored and the length of storage. For example, fresh-picked corn will store better than corn that has been in the market for a few days; a tightly folded inside cereal box liner will prevent a ready-to-eat cereal from becoming limp. The recommended storage time takes these factors into consideration.

Since bacteria frequently get into food through careless food handling, keep everything — hands, pantry, shelves and storage containers — clean.

Selection guidelines

To help assure quality, some products have "open dates" on the package. Product dating is optional on most products. Dates may also be "coded" by the manufacturer and only understood by them. The most commonly used open dates are :

Sell-by Date — This is the last recommended day of sale. The date allows for home storage and use. You will find the date after the statement "sell by (a date)." Breads and baked goods may have "sell-by" dates.

Use-by Date — Tells how long the product will retain top quality after you buy it. You will find this date after statement "Use by." Some packaged goods have "use-by" dates.

Expiration Date — This is the last day the product should be used or eaten. You may find this date after the statement, "Do not use after (date)." Yeast and baking powder have expiration dates.

Pack Date — Canned or packaged foods may have pack dates, which tell you when the product was processed. This does not tell you how long the food will be good.

These are guidelines; if a food is not properly handled, its storage life will be shortened. Follow these tips for purchasing top-quality foods that have been handled safely.

Look for packages of food that are not torn or broken.

Canned goods should be free of dents, cracks and bulging lids.

Refrigerated food should feel cold and frozen food should be frozen solid. Purchase these foods last.

When shopping, place packaged raw meat, poultry and fish in plastic bags and keep from contact with other foods.

Take perishable foods home quickly to refrigerate. If travel time will exceed one hour, pack fresh meats in a cooler with ice and keep in the passenger area of the car in warm weather.

At home, refrigerate perishable food immediately. The "DANGER ZONE" for most food is 40 to 140°F. Bacteria grow most rapidly in this range of temperatures, doubling in number in as little as 20 minutes.

Storage Guidelines

For best results in maintaining product quality practice the rule, FIRST IN, FIRST OUT. This means you use the oldest products first and the newest products later. A good practice in the home is to place the newly purchased products in back of the same products already on the shelf. It may help to write purchase dates on products without "open dates" on the package. Follow recommended storage times for the refrigerator, freezer and pantry.

Freezer

Keep freezer temperature at or below 0°F. A good indication of proper temperature is that ice cream will be frozen solid.

Use moisture-proof, freezer-weight wrap. Examples are foil, freezer bags and freezer paper. Label and date all packages.

Food stored beyond the recommended time will be safe to eat, but eating quality (flavor and texture) and nutritive value will be reduced.

Keep an inventory of freezer contents.

Refrigerator

Use a thermometer to check temperature; it must be between 34°F and 40°F at all times. Avoid frequently opening the refrigerator door, especially in hot weather.

Wrapping perishable food prevents the loss of flavor and the mixing of flavor and odors resulting in, for example, onion-flavored milk.

Raw meat and poultry should be wrapped securely so they do not leak and contaminate other foods. Place the store packages in a plastic bag or place the package on a plate to contain any juices. Clean up leaks with warm soapy water and sanitize with a solution of 1 teaspoon chlorine bleach to 1 quart water.

Cooked meats and leftovers should be tightly wrapped to prevent leakage and drying out.

Pantry :

Storage cabinets should be cool and dry. Storage areas near oven ranges, hot water pipes or heating ducts should not be used because heat and moisture can cause a food to lose its quality more rapidly.

High temperature or humidity may reduce storage time considerably.

Insect infestation can occur in any home. Susceptible foods include cereals, flour, seeds, baking mixes, spices, candy, dried fruits and dry pet foods. Avoid purchasing damaged packages of foods and keep cupboard shelves clean. Storing food in tightly sealed glass, metal or rigid plastic containers may help.

Pantry foods will probably be safe beyond recommended storage time, but eating quality (flavor and texture) and nutritive value will be reduced.

Times for Refrigerator and Freezer Food Storage
Refrigerator and freezer foods

Dairy— Fresh Milk 5-7 days*Buttermilk 1-2 weeks*Canned milk (opened)3-5 days*Yogurt, cottage cheese 7 days*Hard cheese 6-12 weeks 6-12 months Cheese spreads 3-4 weeks*Ice cream*2 month

Eggs— Fresh in shell3 weeks*Hard-cooked1 week*

Meats— fresh Beef roasts, steaks 3-5 days 6-12 months Ground beef or stew 1-2 days 3-4 months Pork roasts, chops 3-5 days 4-6 monthsSausage 1-2 days 1-2 months Chicken or turkey 1-2 days 9-12 months.

Meats— cooked Smoked sausage, whole ham (fully cooked) 7 days 1-2 month sham slices (fully cooked) 3-4 days 1-2 months Hot dogs, luncheon meats (unopened) 2 weeks 1-2 months Hot dogs, luncheon meats (opened) 3-7 days 1-2 months Cooked, leftover meat 3-4 days 2-3 months Leftover gravy and meat broth 1-2 days 2-3 months Cooked, leftover poultry 3-4 days 4-6 months

Seafood— Fresh lean fish: cod, flounder, trout, haddock, halibut, Pollack, perch 1-2 days 4-6 months Fresh fatty fish: mullet, smelt, salmon, mackerel, bluefish, tuna, swordfish 1-2 days 2-3 months Live crabs and lobster same day purchased*Live mussels and clams 2-3 days*Live oysters 7-10 days*Mussels and clams, freshly shucked 1-2 days 3-4 months Oysters, freshly shucked 5-7 days 3-4 months Scallops, crabmeat, shrimp 2-3 days 3-4 months.

Fruits and Vegetables—Apples 1 months 8-12 months Apricots, avocados, grapes, peaches, pears, plums 3-5 days 8-12 months Berries, cherries 2-3 days 8-12 months Grapefruit, lemons, limes, oranges 2 weeks 4-6 months Pineapple 2-3 days 4-6 months Beets, carrots 2 weeks 8-12 months Beans, broccoli, greens, peas, summer squash 3-5 days 8-12 months Celery, cabbage, chilies, lettuce, peppers, tomatoes 1 week 8-12 months Mushrooms 1-2 days 8-12 months.

Pies— Chiffon pie, pumpkin pie 1-2 days 1 month Fruit pie 1-2 days 1 year* Storage here not recommended due to safety or quality issues.

Food Stored in Cool, Dry Place(65 - 70°F)

Canned fruits, tomatoes, pickles 12-18 month scanned meats and vegetables 2-5 years Home-canned foods 1 year Fresh root vegetables (onions, potatoes) 1 week at room temperature or 1-3 months at 45???50? F.

Foods Stored in the Tightly Sealed or Airtight Containers

Staples—Nonfat dry milk 1 year Pasta 1-2 years Rice 1 year Shortening 2 years Sugar, granulated indefinitely Sugar, brown or powdered 18 months Vegetable oil 1 year White flour 10-15 months Whole wheat flour 3 months (best in refrigerator or freezer)Wild rice 6 months.

Packaged Foods— Baking mix (biscuit, cake) 6 months Cereals 12 months.

Dried Foods— Dried apricots 3 months (refrigerate after opening) Dried prunes, raisins 9 months (refrigerate after opening) Dried peas and beans 1 year.

Herbs, Spices and Condiments— Salt, cream of tartaric definitely Ground spices and herbs 2-3 years Whole spices 4-5 years Tabasco, vinegar, Worcestershire sauce 30 months.

Beverages — Bottled water 2-5 yearsJuices 12-18 months Soft drinks 8 months.

Miscellaneous—Chocolate 2 years Chocolate chips, cocoa 18 months Coffee (canned) 12 months Nuts (unshelled) 6-12 months Peanut butter 3-4 months (best refrigerated) Tapioca 4 years Tea 18 months.

Bread and cakes—Store breads and cakes at room temperature. Storing in the refrigerator promotes staling. Use within 3-7 days or freeze.

13
Handling of Food

Food safety has made headlines in newspapers and magazines lately due to outbreaks of diseases such as hepatitis, E.Coli infections, and food poisoning, to name a few. Common food poisonings found in humans include E.coli 0157:H7, salmonella, campylobacter and listeria. Leaving fresh food and water in the bird's cage for several hours may be the cause of bacterial infections in birds.

In our aviary, wet food is left in cages for approximately 6 hours during the winter months, and for less time during the summer months. We try to maintain a temperature in our aviaries of 70°F. but it sometimes rises when the outside temperature is above 90°F. However, we seldom have bacterial problems in our flock.

There are several ways to prepare foods which will help reduce the risk of infectious disease problems in birds :

Wash Your Hands

My veterinarian has told me on more than one occasion that one would be surprised at how effective hand washing with a good antibacterial soap can be against bacteria. I wash my hands several times during preparation of foods for our birds, and especially after handling raw meats or eggs. Hands should be dried with a clean towel or paper towel.

Sanitize Cutting Surfaces and Utensils.

We chop vegetables and fruits with a very sharp knife, on a built-in cutting board, both of which are washed and dried thoroughly between foods.

It would be wise to disinfect your cutting surface and utensils daily with a disinfectant, or a mixture of 3 teaspoons of chlorine bleach mixed in 1 gallon of water. (I don't suggest using this bleach mixture around your birds, however, because it may cause eye and lung irritation). Disinfecting is a sanitation practice that is absolutely necessary if raw meat or eggs have been cut on the cutting surface.

Wash Foods

Before foods are cut and served, they are thoroughly washed. Some people use a solution of 1 part Nolvansan liquid to 8 parts water; or 1 teaspoon chlorine bleach (which contains sodium hypochlorite and no phosphorous) in 1 gallon of water. Fruits and vegetables can be soaked for up to 10 minutes, then rinsed thoroughly in another bowl with running water for at least 5 minutes. Be sure to inspect foods thoroughly before washing them to detect mold, overripe or brown spots.

It should go without saying that any meats which are being prepared should be thoroughly washed, whether they are for human or your birds' consumption.

Cook Meats Thoroughly

Any meats we serve our birds, which include turkey, chicken, or beef, must be well cooked.

One caller told me she feeds her birds meats prepared on the barbeque grill cooked medium well-done. I would strongly suggest that if you want to serve ground meat cooked on the grill, to re cook it in the microwave, to make absolutely certain the center is well cooked. (Note: Cooking the center to well done is applicable only to ground meat. The center of a steak or roast is absolutely free of E. coli or other contaminants. Only something the animal consumes can get into the meat or something live which infiltrates, such as trichinosis in pork.

Also, remember that meats should not be served to our birds if they have been left out for any length of time. A good example of this would be turkey that has been left on the table after Thanksgiving dinner, while the participants are visiting.

Of course, food handling is not always the cause of infectious agents found in foods. The E.coli bacterium was found in frozen hamburger patties prepared at a meat plant. An outbreak of hepatitis A was traced to strawberries packaged by a company in San Diego, but the frozen strawberries were from Mexico, and used in Michigan. An outbreak of cyclospora (a parasite) was blamed on Guatemalan raspberries.

Though not affecting our birds, another disease outbreak was caused by tainted ice cream which had been transported by trucks that previously carried raw eggs.

A recent newspaper article reported that on crops, contamination occurs from the use of untreated water for irrigation or fertilizers containing the dangerous organisms. It went on to say that cattle feed may include contaminated animal parts or waste material. It was further reported that Mexico is the primary exporter of vegetables to the United States. The author of this article explained that in one particular town whose crops he observed, the surrounding communities emptied their sewage into the river which supplied the water to irrigate fields of corn.

Mexico is now shipping winter fruits and vegetables which may be contaminated with pesticides or other chemicals. Restrictions on chemicals sprayed on crops are much less stringent south of the border than in the United States. Some foods coming in are hot peppers, watermelons, squash, strawberries, carrots, berries, kiwi, other tropical fruits, and pears. It is a good idea to check packages or signs at the produce counters in grocery stores before purchasing fresh fruits and vegetables. In the past, imported grapes have received bad press due to overuse of chemicals.

Organically grown and prepared foods are very popular for ourselves and our birds, but they are expensive and may be difficult to grow ourselves. Besides, their safety has been questioned because they are often fertilized with manure which could well be contaminated.

Unfortunately, the federal agencies and watchdog groupcannot be expected to inspect and approve every fruit and vegetable we and our birds eat, so it is up to us to determine which foods are safe and healthy, and to educate ourselves about safe food preparation, for the benefit of ourselves and our wards.

14
Food Groups

Basic Food Groups

Food should be evaluated for their total contribution of nutrients and not in terms of one on two nutrients. A diet in evaluated in terms of the contribution of its nutrients and how far these nutrients meet the body requirements of an individual.

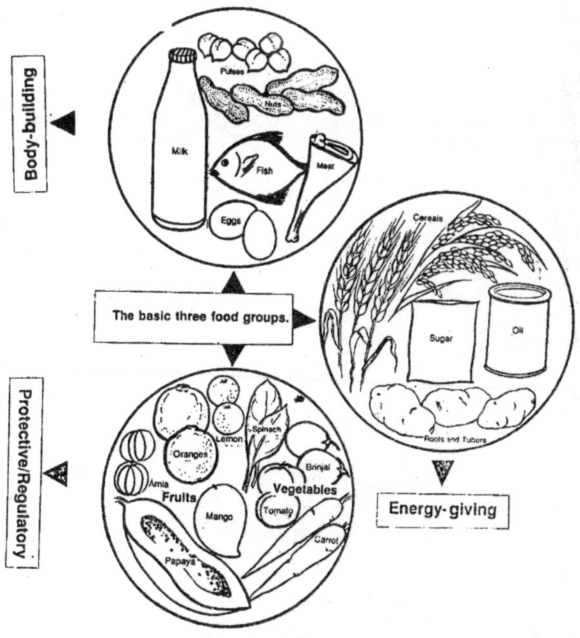

Classification of food groups.

The quality and quantity of food stuffs in the diet of people varieties according to their age, sex and occupation. For example a baby needs much less food than a school child.

The determine the nutrients requirement of a body, its is important to understand what balanced diet is, to require the contribution of each food groups to the total nutrition content of the diet and the basic dietary patterns laid down for an individual.

A balanced diet is defined as one which contains different types of foods in such quantities and proportions that the need for calories, minerals, vitamins, and other nutrients is adequate met. A small provision has to be made for extra nutrients to withstand short durations of leanness. The diagram shows how a balanced diet may be based on various of food derived from each of the food groups indicated.

The diagram indicates total food groups.

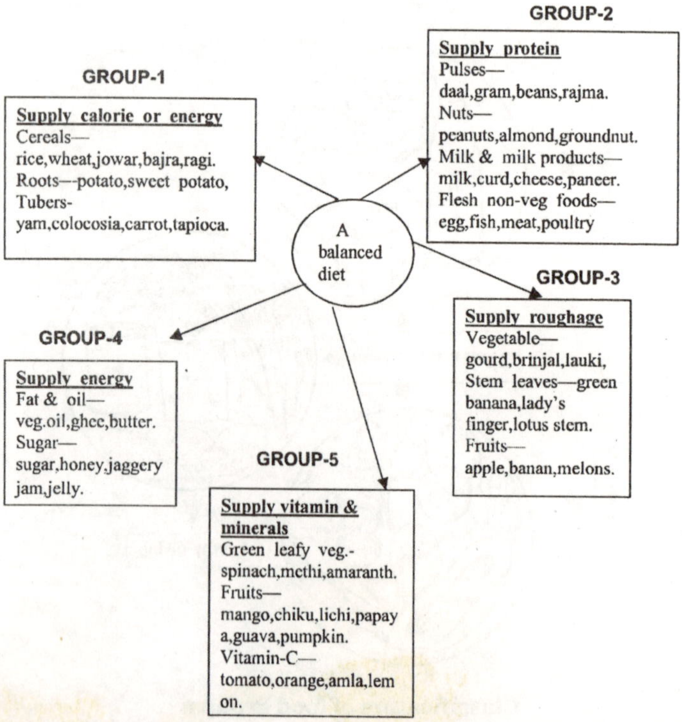

The Five Major Food Groups

A well-balanced diet offers you many mouth-watering food choices. With this helpful guide, you'll learn about AHA-recommended servings and sizes for each food group or specialized category. You'll also see how easy and fun it is to combine a wide variety of foods to create a well-balanced diet.

Each of the basic food groups supplies a different combination of nutrients, vitamins and minerals. Let caloric needs and a healthy appetite be your guide. But remember, variety is the key to good nutrition.

Group-I (Cereals, Roots and Tubers, Bread, Rice, and Pasta)

These are all primarily supply energy on calories. Example of these food groups are rice, wheat, Jowar, Bajra, ragi, and other cereals, taioca, Potatoes, sweet potato, arvi and yam are examples of roots and tubers.

A significant contribution towards calories, proteins, iron and vitamins in made by this group. These foods are cheap and are taken in large amounts their importance in law income group diets. This food groups ranks as an important source of thiamine, niacim and iron.

The main cereals consumed in India are rice, wheat and millets (Jowar, bajra, ragi etc). They are the cheapest sources of calories. In view of the large amounts in which cereals are included in the diet, they form important sources of nutrients in an average Indian diet. The seed or the kennel of the cereal grain is divided into three parts, the bran, the germs and the endosperm. Cereal very some what some what in composition, the average percentage composition of the whole fresh in: Protein 12 per cent, Fat 2 per cent, Carbohydrates 75 per cent, Water 10 per cent, Minerals and vitamins 1 per cent.

Grain products like bread, cereal, rice, and pasta are good for you. They are important sources of vitamins and minerals. Breads, cereals, rice, and pasta are also good sources of carbohydrates like starch and fiber.

Many people think that starchy foods like breads, rice and pasta are fattening. They are not. But when you add fats like margarine, oil, mayonnaise, cheese sauce or gravy to them, you add many extra calories.

Whole-grain foods have more fiber than white grain foods. There are many kinds of whole-grain foods, such as oatmeal, brown rice, grits, corn tortillas and whole wheat bread. You may want to try a whole grain bread instead of white bread. Use brown rice instead of white rice or mix them together the next time you have rice.

Some breads and cereals have lots of fat and sugar added when they are manufactured. Croissants, Danish, doughnuts, cake and some muffins have more fat and calories than servings of plain breads and cereals. If you enjoy sweet breads and cereals, you don't have to give them up. Try eating these foods less often or in small amounts. When you shop, read the food labels and look for breads, cereals, rice and pasta mixes that have less fat and sugar in them. You can also cut down on fat when you make rice or pasta dishes. Try using less oil, butter, or margarine than the recipe says. Sometimes you can cut the fat in half without changing the way the food tastes or looks!

Group-II (Protein giving foods- Meat, Poultry, Fish, Dry Beans, Eggs, Milk, Yogurt, and Cheese and Nuts)

The food stuffs in this group are primarily sources of protein, through cereals also furnish protein. Daals, grains, peas, beans, groundnuts, cashew nuts, almons, coconuts, milk, card, buttermilk, paneer, cheese, khoya, eggs, fish, mutton, chicken, pork and other flesh foods make up their groups. It provides protein both from the vegetable and animal. Milk and dairy products are important sources of calcium and riboflavin.

This group comprises of food stuffs which contain mostly protein, but in widely varying amounts. Animal foods, such as meet, fish, eggs are rich sources of protein. Among vegetable foods pulses to nuts are the richest sources of protein with amounts often exceeding these resent in animal foods. Soya beans in unique contains over 40 per cent of protein.

Vegetable Protein. Pulses is a terms which includes daals and grams. These are really important in the diet as sources of proteins because flesh foods are consumed only in small amounts.

Pulse proteins are biological value because of the deficiency of an amino-acid, methi onion. Red gram is also deficient in tryptophane. However, pulse proteins are rich in lysine and they are, therefore good supplementary value to cereal diets. Cysine deficit in cereals is made food by lysine present in pulses and thus the overall biological value of the cereal pulse diet is better. Pulses can not be rich sources of mineral but rich in vitamins of B group i.e. folic acid and thiamine. Nuts and oil seeds are rich in protein, contain al and good sources of calories. Groundnuts is a rich source of B complex vitamin group.

Animal Protein. Milk serves as the sole food of the young during the most critical period of life. Milk is used as food for various mammals. Milk products include cheese, khoya, rabri and curd. Milk contains essential amino acids which needs for tissue synthesis. Milk sugar or lactose is a carbohydrate which favors the absorb of calcium and phosphorous and the synthesis of same B complex vitamins in the intestine. Milk supply cereals minerals, milk is an outstanding sources of riboflavin, vitamin A, vitamin B.

Curd. Curd contains lactic acid bacteria which causes fermentation and set the milk. Nutrients Present in milk remain in the curd, it is very easily digested.

Cheese. Protein in cheese contain all the essential amino acids and are biological value. Lactose present in milk remains in the cheese. Calcium, thiamine and riboflavin are last during proportion.

Egg. It is an excellent sources of protein. It contains highest quality of protein, fat, vitamin A and B, iron, phosphorous, calcium etc. Food preparation destroy the both Avider and inhibitor.

Fish, Meat, Poultry. This group is the master sources of cholesterol in diet. This lipid is not uniformly present in all flesh foods, brain and shall fish are the riches sources of it. These foods are high in sodium, B-complex vitamins, and less sources of calcium and vitamins.

Meat, poultry, fish, dry beans, eggs, and nuts are important sources of protein, iron, zinc, and B vitamins. This group includes plant foods and animal foods.

Some meats and meat products are high in fat. There are many ways to reduce the fat you get from these meats. You can choose leaner cuts like chuck, bottom round or top round of beef, pork loin or lamb shank. You can trim fat from meat before cooking and eating. You can take the skin off chicken. Many processed meats like hot dogs, sausage, pepperoni, bacon, ham and luncheon meats are high in fat and sodium. If you enjoy eating these meats, try having them less often and when you do, try eating them in smaller amounts.

Because eggs are a good source of iron and protein, they are counted as a meat serving. Most of the fat in eggs is found in the yolk. When you use the egg whites, you can cut the fat and keep the protein and vitamins you need.

Plant foods like lentils, black-eyed peas, chick peas and other dried beans and peas are inexpensive sources of protein. Unlike meats, beans are low in fat and high in fiber. Nuts and nut butters like peanuts and peanut butter are good sources of protein and iron; but they are higher in fat than other plant foods.

You can get the nutrients you need from this group without a lot of fat and without costing a lot. Many lean meats like beef chuck are also lower in cost. If you buy ground beef that is 70 per cent fat because it is less expensive, you can still reduce the fat. Try draining the meat after you cook it or add other ingredients. Mix small amounts of meat with pasta, beans and rice to stretch your food dollar. You will get the same nutrients but it will cost you less.

Milk and foods made from milk are the best sources of the mineral calcium. They also provide us with vitamin A, protein and phosphorus. Fortified milk has vitamin D added to it.

The foods in this group are important because all of the nutrients work together to keep our bones strong and healthy. It may be difficult to get enough calcium unless we include these foods in our diets. We can make sure we get the milk and calcium we need by making puddings and soups with milk.

Some milk products like ice cream, cheese, whole milk and foods made from whole milk are high in fat. We can choose low-fat or skim milk products, like low-fat yogurt, skim milk and low-fat cheeses to keep the fat in our diets down.

Some people who have problems digesting milk products because of lactose (sugar) in milk. Today there are many lactose-free products to try.

Group III:-(Fats, Oils, Sugar, Jaggery and Sweets)

These food stuffs supply energy ore calories-veg. Oils, Vanaspati, ghee, butter, cream, sugar, Jaggery. This food group constitutes about $1/6^{th}$ of the energy value of the diet, but not add to protein, minerals, ore vitamins. Oils adds in diet to increase taste, flavor and colour in food. Commonly available cooking oils are mustered oil, coconut oil, ground nut oil, palm oil and sunflower oil.

Visible fats which are available in diet are butt, ghee, vegetable oil, vanaspati and hydo generated oil. Fats are also sources of energy. Butter, margarine, hydrogenated fats contain saturated fatty acids. Vegetable oil whereas contains or rich in Polyunsaturated fatty acid in diet. Sugar and Jaggary are as sweetening agent in beverages. They are pure sources of energy. Jaggery, sugar and honey are also source of iron.

Fats, oils and sweets give us calories. Fats and oils like salad dressings, mayonnaise, butter, margarine and lard tend to be high in calories because of the fat they contain. Sweets like candy, soft drinks, syrups, jams, and jellies are made mostly of sugars. Most of these foods do not contain many vitamins or minerals. So they are called "empty calorie" foods.

Fats, oils and sweets are not bad foods. When we eat them along with foods like grains, fruits, vegetables, milk and meat products they are part of a healthy diet. Eating too many fats, oils or sweets can be a problem when we eat them instead of foods and nutrients we get in the other food groups.

Fats, oils and sweets add flavor and variety to our diets. We don't have to give them up. We can use less of them to help us stay fit and healthy. We can spread a smaller amount of butter, margarine or jelly on toast or muffins. We can use less fat and oil in cooking. When we cook we can cut down of some of the fats and sugars by reducing the amounts of these ingredients in the recipes we make.

Group-IV:- Protective(Vegetable and Fruits)

These group mainly sources of mineral and vitamins.

(A) Green leafy vegetables – Palak, methi, arvi, Kulfa and other leafy veg.

(B) Yellow and orange fruits – Papaya, mango, carrot, yellow pumpkin.

(C) Fruits and vegetables rich in vitamin C – Amla, guava, lemon, orange, phalsa.

They are mainly rich sources of ascorbic acid, vitamin A, 1/5th of iron etc.

Green leafy vegetables are rich source of carotene, vitamin C, riboflavin, folic acid, calcium and iron, which are essential fore growth and maintenance of normal health. Deep yellow and orange coloured fruits and vegetables are high source of carotene, B complex vitamins, etc. citrus fruits like lemon lime, Alma, falsa, etc rich in vitamin A-C, which in sugar, vitamin B, and B_2, starch.

Fruits are important sources of vitamins and carbohydrates like fiber and sugar. They are low in calories and naturally sweet. Fruits and their juices are good sources of water, too.

Different fruits contain different vitamins, so it is important to eat a variety of fruits. Mangoes, papayas, melons and citrus fruits, like oranges and grapefruit, are high in vitamin C. Cantaloupe, apricots, peaches, and nectarines are sources of vitamin A.

Whole fruits like apples and grapes contain more fiber than fruit juices and sauces, like applesauce and grape juice. Dried fruits like figs, prunes and raisins are good sources of fiber, too. Canned fruits packed in syrup have a lot of added sugar. They are higher in calories than fresh fruits. When you shop for canned fruits, look for fruit that is packed in juice instead of syrup.

Group-V:- Other Vegetables

Vegetables provide variety in taste and texture and furnish roughage in the diet, e.g. fruits, stems, leaves and flowers of plants, lady's finger, brinjal, bitter guard and other guard, cabbage, cauliflower, and drumsticks. These add variety and flavor to food and they supply minerals and vitamins also. The skins, seeds and fibers of fruits and vegetables are also of value in the maintenance of the normal gastrointestinal motility by contributing some indigestible fiber which is useful as roughage.

Vegetables are a source of important vitamins, minerals and carbohydrates. Because vegetables differ in the vitamins and minerals they contain, it is important to eat a variety of vegetables. Cabbages, plantains, peppers and leafy green vegetables like poke greens and kale are rich sources of vitamin C. Deep orange and dark green vegetables are high in vitamin A. Broccoli, spinach, collards and kale are dark green vegetables that contain calcium and iron. Cabbage family vegetables like broccoli, cauliflower, turnips and rutabagas help prevent certain cancers.

Fresh vegetables are naturally low in fat, calories and sodium. Extra fat and calories can come from cooking or other types of processing. If you add fat, oil, margarine or lard when you cook vegetables, you also add fat and calories. If you buy frozen vegetables with special sauces, you may also be adding fat and calories. You can buy frozen vegetables without special sauces and get the same nutrients as fresh vegetables. Some canned vegetables have added salt. While the salt adds flavor, it also adds extra sodium to your diet. When you shop for canned vegetables, look for vegetables with no salt added.

Recommended Allowances of Food Group

A balanced diet may be planned depending on the age, sex, and work type done by the individual. In using them, the following points may be kept in mind :-

(1) Dietary allowances for adults are for a reference man, weighing 55 kg and a woman weighting 45 kg. The allowances for calories, protein and B complex vitamins are increased depending on the body weight.

(2) The protein allowances is about 1 gm per body weight per day. For infants, children, pregnant and lactating woman, it is desirable to supply 25 per cent of the total protein fresh animal foods such as milk, egg, fresh food.

(3) Fats requirement is not desirable to have more than 15% of the calories in the diet. About 15 grams of oil present in the diet.

(4) Requirement of carbohydrates are not more than 70 percent of the calories in diet.

(5) Minerals such as magnesium, copper, iodine, are needed in small amounts.

(6) Most of the ingredients of a diet are rich in phosphorus and it is for this reason the allowances for this elements are not listed.

(7) The total vitamin A value of a diet in terms of retinal can be calculated as follows :

Total Vitamin A value as retinal (mg)=Retinal (mg) + â-carotene (mg) 4

(8) Vitamin-D requirement is undoubtedly met by the action of sunlight on the skin. However, it may not be advisable to rely entirely on sunshine for vitamin-D requirements in the children.

Balanced Diet for Adult Man

	Sedentary Work		*Moderate Work*		*Heavy Work*	
	Veg. (gm)	*Non -Veg. (gm)*	*Veg. (gm)*	*Non -Veg. (gm)*	*Veg. (gm)*	*Non. Veg. (gm)*
Cereal	400	400	475	475	650	650
Pulses	70	55	80	65	80	65
g.l. veg.	100	100	125	125	125	125
Veg.	75	75	75	75	100	100
Roots	75	75	100	100	100	100
Fruits	30	30	30	30	30	30
Milk	200	100	200	100	200	100
Fat	35	40	40	40	50	50
Meat	—	30	—	30	—	30
Egg	—	30	—	30	—	30
Sugar	30	30	40	40	55	55
Nuts	—	—	—	—	50	50

* An additional 30 gms of fat and oil can be include in the diet in place of Groundnuts.

Balanced Diet for Adult Woman

	Sedentary Work		*Moderate Work*		*Heavy Work*	
	Veg. (gm)	*Non -Veg. (gm)*	*Veg. (gm)*	*Non -Veg. (gm)*	*Veg. (gm)*	*Non. Veg. (gm)*
Cereal	300	300	350	350	475	475
Pulses	60	45	70	55	70	55
g.l. veg.	125	125	125	125	125	125
Veg.	75	75	75	75	100	100
Roots	50	50	75	75	100	100
Fruits	30	30	30	30	30	30
Milk	200	100	200	100	200	100
Fat	30	35	35	40	45	50
Meat	—	30	—	30	—	30
Egg	—	30	—	30	—	30
Sugar	30	30	30	30	40	40
Nuts	—	—	—	—	40	40

* An additional 25 gms of fat and oil can be include in the diet in place of Groundnuts.

Balanced Diet for Children

	1-3 Years		*4-6 Years*	
	Veg. (gm)	*Non-veg. (gm)*	*Veg. (gm)*	*Non-veg (gm)*
Cereal	150	150	200	200
Pulses	50	40	60	50
G.L. Veg.	50	50	75	75
Veg.	30	30	50	50
Roots	30	30	50	50
Fruits	50	50	50	50
Fat	20	20	25	25
Meat	—	30	—	30
Egg	—	30	—	30
Sugar	30	30	40	40

Balanced Diet for Children

	7-9 Years		*10-12 Years*	
	Veg. (gm)	*Non-veg. (gm)*	*Veg. (gm)*	*Non-veg (gm)*
Cereal	250	250	320	320
Pulses	50	60	70	60
G.L. Veg.	75	75	100	100
Veg.	50	50	75	75
Roots	50	50	75	75
Fruits	50	50	50	50
Fat	20	20	25	25
Meat	—	30	—	30
Egg	—	30	—	30
Sugar	50	50	50	50

Balanced Diet for Children (Boys)

	13-15 Years		*16-18 Years*	
	Veg. (gm)	*Non-veg. (gm)*	*Veg. (gm)*	*Non-veg (gm)*
Cereal	430	430	450	450
Pulses	70	50	70	50
G.L. Veg.	100	100	100	100
Veg.	75	75	75	75
Roots	75	75	100	100
Fruit	30	30	30	30
Milk	250	150	250	150
Fat & Oil	35	40	45	50
Meat	—	30	—	30
Egg	—	30	—	30
Sugar	30	30	40	40
Nuts	—	—	50	50

An additional 30 gms of Fat & Oil can be included in the diet in the place of groundnut.

Balanced Diet for Children (Girls)

	13-15 Years	
	veg. (gm)	*Non-veg (gm)*
Cereal	350	350
Pulses	70	50
G.L. Veg.	150	150
Veg.	75	75
Roots	75	75
Fruit	30	30
Milk	250	150
Fat & Oil	35	40
Meat	—	30
Egg	—	30
Sugar	30	30
Nuts	—	—

An additional 30 gms of Fat & Oil can be included in the diet in the place of groundnut.

Balanced Diet for Adult Woman

	Pregnancy		Lactation	
	Veg. (gm)	*Non-veg. (gm)*	*Veg. (gm)*	*Non-veg (gm)*
Cereal	350	350	400	400
Pulses	60	45	70	55
G.L. Veg.	150	150	150	150
Veg.	75	75	75	75
Roots	50	50	50	50
Fruits	30	30	30	30
Milk	325	225	325	225
Fat & Oil	30	30	30	45
Sugar	40	40	50	50
Meat	—	30	—	30
Nuts	—	—	—	—
Egg	—	30	—	30

Energy Requirements with Different Body Weight (Male Activity)

Body Weight	*BMR*	*Sedentary*	*Moderate*	*Heavy*
40	1225	1960	2328	3063
45	1300	2080	2470	3250
50	1370	2192	2603	3425
55	1445	2312	2746	3612
60	1515	2424	2879	3788
65	1590	2544	3021	3975
70	1660	2656	3154	4150
75	1755	2806	3335	4388

Energy Requirements with Different Body Weight (Female Activity)

Body Weight	*BMR*	*Sedentary*	*Moderate*	*Heavy*
35	960	1536	1824	2400
40	1030	1648	1957	2575
45	1100	1760	2090	2750
50	1170	1872	2223	2925
55	1240	1984	2356	3100
60	1310	2096	2489	3275
65	1380	2208	2622	3450
70	1450	2320	2755	3625

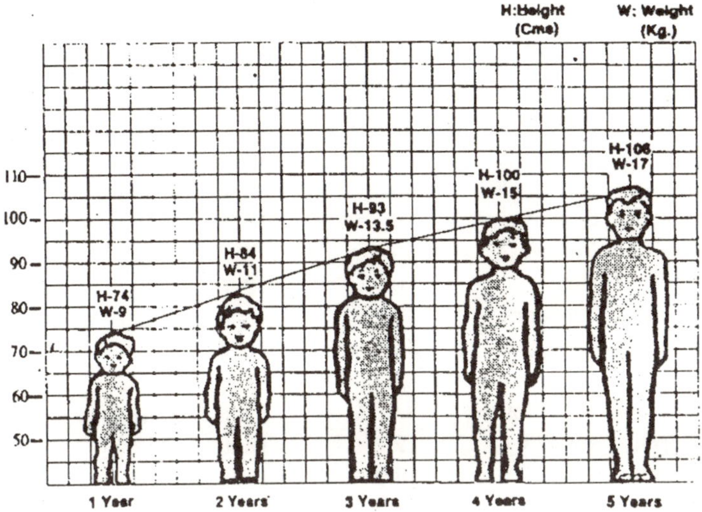

Average Height / Weight of Preschool children.

Height and Weight of Indian Children (Girls)

Age	*Height (Cm)*	*Weight (Kg)*
1	78.0	9.9
2	87.9	11.6
3	96.2	13.7
4	104.1	15.8
5	112.2	18.6
6	117.7	21.5
7	122.6	24.4
8	127.2	25.9
9	133.0	29.8
10	138.9	33.5
11	145.0	37.1
12	150.9	42.9
13	153.4	44.5
14	155.0	46.7
15	155.9	48.7
16	156.0	49.7

Recommended Dietary Allowances for Indians

Group	*Particular (activity)*	*Body Weight (kgs.)*	*Energy (kcal)*	*Protein (gms.)*	*Fat (gms.)*
Men	Sedentary	60	2425	60	20
Men	Moderate	60	2875	60	20
Men	Heavy	60	3800	60	20
Women	Sedentary	50	1875	50	20
Women	Moderate	50	2225	50	20
Women	Heavy	50	2925	50	20
Women	Pregnant	50	+300	+15	+10
Women	Lactation	50	+550	+25	+15
Infant	0-6 Months	5.4	108	2.05	—
Infant	6-12 Months	8.6	98	1.65	—
Children	1-3 Yrs	12.2	1240	22	25
Children	4-6 Yrs	19.0	1690	30	25
Children	7-9 Yrs	26.9	1940	41	25
Boys	10-12 Yrs	35.4	2190	54	22
Boys	13-15 Yrs	47.8	2060	65	22
Boys	16-18 Yrs	57.1	2640	78	22
Girls	10-12 Yrs	31.5	1970	57	22
Girls	13-15 Yrs	46.7	2450	70	22
Girls	16-18 Yrs	49.9	2060	63	22

Daily Requirements of Food Groups

Everyone wants to know how much they should eat to stay healthy. It's a tricky question, though. It depends on your age, whether you're a girl or a boy, and how active you are. Kids who are more active burn more calories so they need more calories. But we can give you some estimates for how much you need of each food group.

Grains

Grains are measured out in ounce equivalents. What the heck are they? Ounce equivalents are just another way of showing a serving size.

Here are ounce equivalents for common grain foods. An ounce equivalent equals :

1 piece of bread

1/2 cup of cooked cereal, like oatmeal

1/2 cup of rice or pasta

1 cup of cold cereal

4- to 8-year-olds need 4 to 5 ounce equivalents each day.

9- to 13-year-old girls need 5 ounce equivalents each day.

9- to 13-year-old boys need 6 ounce equivalents each day.

And one last thing about grains: Try to eat a lot of whole grains, such as 100% wheat bread, brown rice, and oatmeal.

Vegetables

Of course, you need your vegetables, especially those dark green and orange ones. But how much is enough? Vegetable servings are measured in cups.

4- to 8-year-olds need 1 1/2 cups of veggies each day.

9- to 13-year-old girls need 2 cups of veggies each day.

9- to 13-year-old boys need 2 1/2 cups of veggies each day.

Fruits

Sweet, juicy fruit is definitely part of a healthy diet. Here's how much you need :

4- to 8-year-olds need 1 cup to 1 1/2 cups of fruit each day.

9- to 13-year-old girls need 1 1/2 cups of fruit each day.

9- to 13-year-old boys need 1 1/2 cups of fruit each day.

Milk and Other Calcium-Rich Foods

Calcium builds strong bones to last a lifetime, so you need these foods in your diet.

4- to 8-year-olds need 1 cup to 2 cups of milk (or another calcium-rich food) each day.

9- to 13-year-old girls need 3 cups of milk (or another calcium-rich food) each day.

9- to 13-year-old boys need 3 cups of milk (or another calcium-rich food) each day.

If you want something other than milk, you can substitute yogurt, cheese, or calcium-fortified orange juice - just to name a few.

Meats, Beans, Fish, and Nuts

These foods contain iron and lots of other important nutrients. Like grains, these foods are measured in ounce equivalents.

An ounce equivalent of this group would be :

1 ounce of meat, poultry, or fish

1/4 cup cooked dry beans

1 egg

1 tablespoon of peanut butter a small handful of nuts or seeds

4- to 8-year-olds need 3 to 4 ounce equivalents each day.

9- to 13-year-old girls need 5 ounce equivalents each day.

9- to 13-year-old boys need 5 ounce equivalents each day.

Whoa! That's a lot to swallow. The good news is that your mom, dad, and the other grownups in your life will help you eat what you need to stay healthy. There's more good news - you don't have to become a perfect eater overnight. Just remember those stairs climbing up the side of the new pyramid and take it one step at a time.

15
Balanced Diet

Adequate nutrient is a vital need for energy one, of all ages. However, Some groups are more Prone to Mal nutrient than others on account of various factors. For example, young children are adolescent boys and girls, expectant mothers and nursing mothers have increased demands for nutrients, this is because young children and adolescent individuals are in a period of rapid growth, the pregnant woman need to nourish the growing fetus.

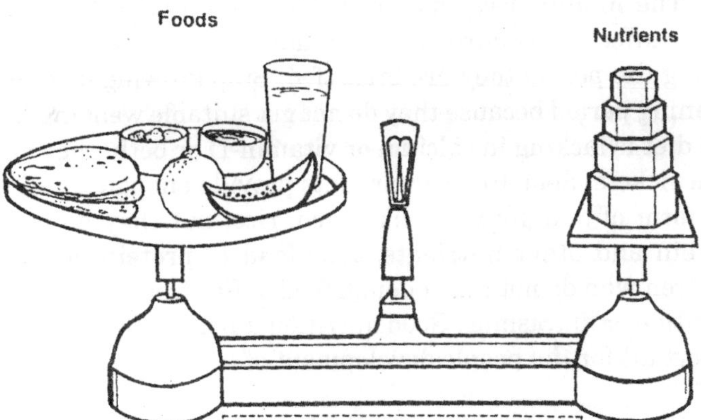

Different foods in the right amounts and proportions provide all essential nutrients and hence make a balanced diet

Nursing mothers nourish their growing infants, they have increased nutritional requirements. Increased requirements for specific nutrients occur at other stages too – a child needs more calcium in relation to its energy intake than the adults. It is necessary to consume adequate amounts of a variety of foods so as to provide all the nutrients required.

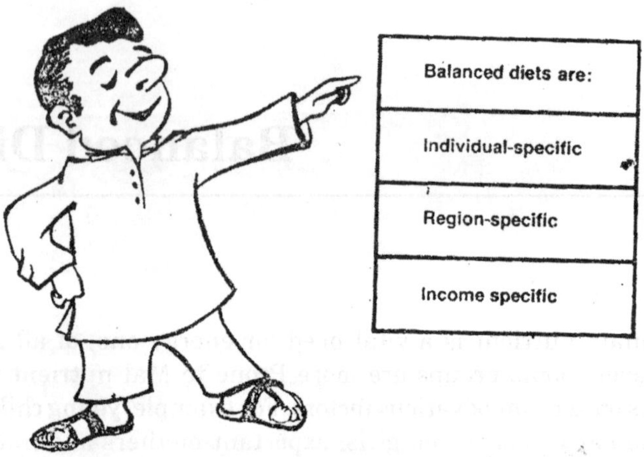

Prefer Balanced Diet.

Diet for infants

The infants doest not get adequate nutrition, its growth will be affected. Children in poor families who grow satisfaction during the period they are breastfed. Stop growing during the meaning period because they do not get suitable weaving foods. The diet is lacking in calcium or vitamin-D or both, they suffer from rickets. Sometimes their diets provide enough calories in the form of starchy foods like sago, rice, but they do not get protein and other nutrients. This lead to protein deficiency children who do not take enough food suffer from severe under nutrition or marasmus. Good nutrition during childhood is very important for the people development of the child.

Weaning is a process in which an infant's diet pattern is gradually changed from liquid foods like breast milk and suitable milk and food. This process can be started from the age of 3 to 4 months.

Diet for new born —

The best food for the new born baby is mother's milk. Poorly nourished mother is able to nurse her child satisfactorily at least

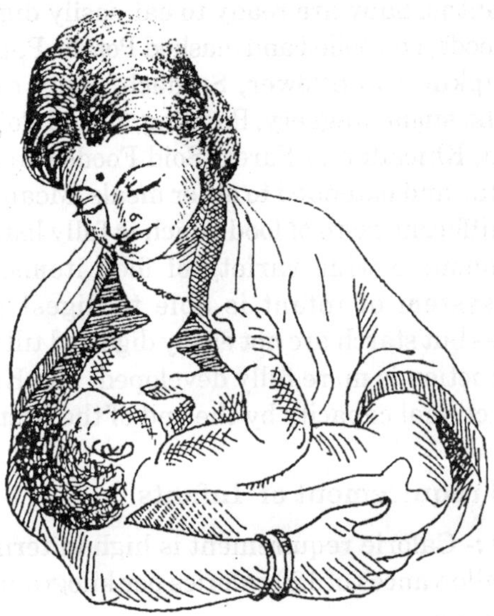

Importance of Breast Milk.

the first few months of life. Carbohydrates, fat, proteins and minerals contents of breast milk are not seriously affected by the diet of the mother under ordinary conditions. Under normal condition deficiency disease such as infantile scurvy or rickets are not found in breast fed babies.

Breast milk free from contamination and adulteration and supply all nutrients in people balance amount which needed for body. Breast milk contains in memo-Protein which protects the child to save infection. Well nourished baby doubles his birth weight by 3 to 4 months of age. Human breast milk provides ascorbic acid to avoid deficiency system of malnutrition.

Diet for weaning

Baby start weaning diets with cereals foods provided the food is cooked soft and mashed to a thin consistency. Non-starch foods, soups, creamy mashed vegetables, mashed fruits may be gradually start during the meaning stage. Fruits and vegetables correct the deficiency of iron and vitamin C, which is present in human milk.

At 6 months, baby are ready to eat easily digestable solid and starchy foods, i.e., boiled and mashed Potato, Papaya, Orange, Carrot, Pumpkin, Cauliflower, Spinach. Baby can eat fruits cooked in milk, sugar, Jaggery, Pudding, Baked Potatoes, Sweet Potato, Dalia, Khichdi and Farex. Soid Foods can be first start with lunchtime and extended to other meals. Meaning helps the child to get different taste of food which is fully leaned the child is able to consume wide variety of food items. The gastro infestional system of infant is able to digest protein, fat, carbohydrates but starch are not easily digested till the digestive enzyme production is more fully developed. The Kidneys reach their full functional capacity by the end of the first year.

Nutritional requirement of Infants

Energy :- Calorie requirement is high in term of his body weight. The allowances of 120 calories per kilogram body weight for the infant, i.e.

Basal metabolism	-	60 calories
Dynamic Action	-	5 calories
Growth	-	15 calories
Faecal loss	-	5 calories
Activity	-	35 calories

Protein. When a regular mixed diet is given the allowance should be increased, i.e., 2.9 gm. per kilogram body weight from six months to 1 year.

Fat. Fat is important to maintain calories adequate. About 3 per cent of total calorie intake should be supplied as linoleic acid, to maintain the integrity of the skin and normal growth. Human milk supply about 6-9 per cent of calories as linolate.

Water. Daily turnover of water by the infant is as much as 15 percent of his body weight.

Minerals. The Sodium requirement about 1 mg per kilogram.

Vitamin :- The vitamin-D requirement is about 400 I.U.

Recommended Allowances

Calories	-	900-1000
Protein	-	17 gm
Calcium	-	0.4 to 0.5 gm.
Iron	-	15 mg.

Weaning Diet for Infants (4-12 Months)

4-6 Months -	Fruit juice with sugar light soups
5-6 Months -	Cereals cooked in water milk Soup
6-7 Months -	Egg Yellow Mashed Banana Potato with milk Boiled fruits with milk
7-8 Months -	Khichri Well Cooked Vegetable
10-12 Month -	Soft boiled Egg Scrambled Egg light custard boiled meat

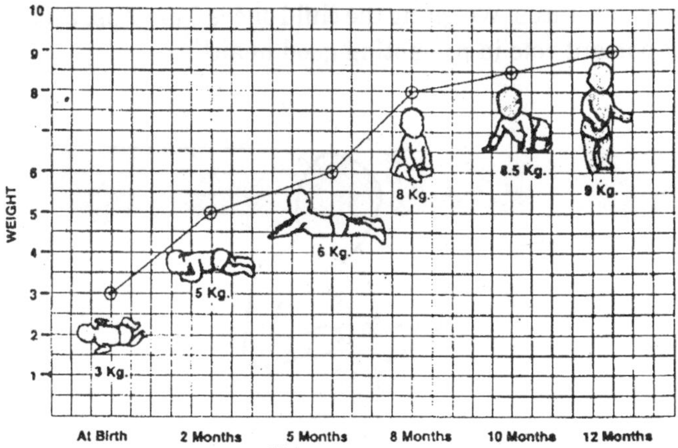

Average body weight of Infants from birth to twelve months.

Weaning daily Diet plan for Infants (4-12 Months)

EM	-	Breast Milk
BF	-	Half Boiled Egg Yellow
MD	-	Cow's Milk

Noon	-	Mixed Vegetable Soup
Lunch	-	Orange juice with Sugar
Afternoon	-	Cow's Milk
EV	-	Skimmed Curd
DIN	-	Spinach Khichri
BT	-	Breast Milk

Diet for Preschool Child

Child is the age of 1-6 years group as a preschool child. From the growth development side the preschool child is different from infant. A preschool grows rapidly, but compared to infancy the rate of growth is slower and more gradual at this stage. The average weight gain is about 2-2.5 kg each year. Preschool gains height than weight. By the three years the child is about 93 cm–100 cm. Preschooler is increased physical activity regular weight gain is the most important sign of the child's overall health and nutritional status. Weighing the child one is 3 months. Diet plays an important role in promoting good health.

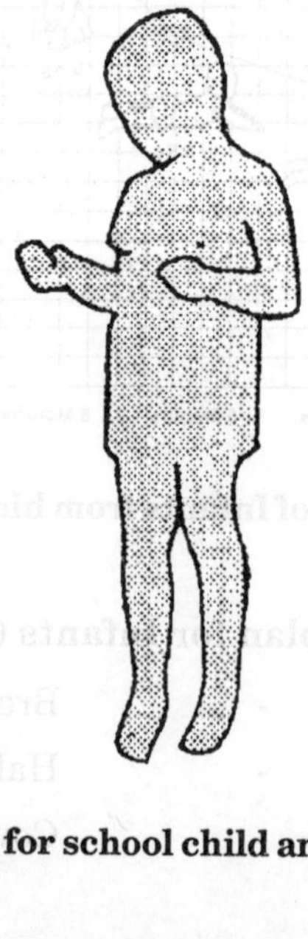

Meal Planning for school child and adolescend.

Preschool years represent age about 1-6 years At this stage need of nutrients very depending on the level of growth and physical activity.

Energy requirement of preschool child increases with age, other nutrients also high but need for a few nutrients like protein, calcium, vitamins and iron is most, because these support the growth and development. The diet of the preschooler must provide sufficient amount of vitamin A and Iron.

Recommended Dietary Intake

Nutrients	*RDI* *1-3 years*	*Age group* *4-6 years*
Energy	1240	1690
Protein	22	30
Calcium	400	400
Iron	12	18
Vitamin A	400	400
Thiamine	0.6	0.9
Riboflavin	0.7	1.0
Folic Acid	30	40

Recommended Allowance

Calories	-	1200 kcal
Protein	-	20 gm
Calcium	-	0.4-0.5 gm
Vitamin-A	-	1000

Diet for Infants (1-2 Yrs)

Early Morning	Milk-1Glass
Break Fast	Scrambled Egg-1no.
	Toast-1 slice
Mid Morning	Orange/Mossambi juice-1Glass
Lunch	Vegetable Pulao-1Katori
	Bhoondi Raita-1Katori

Evening	Milk-1Glass
	Biscuit-2nos.
Dinner	Mixed Pulse and Vegetable-1Katori
	Vegetable. Soup-1Bowl
	Bread-1Slice
	Salad-1Plate
Bed Time	Ice Cream-1/2Katori

Diet for Infants (3 Yrs)

Early Morning	Milk-1 Glass
	Apple-1no
Break Fast	Sweet Dalia-1 Katori
Mid Morning	Orange juice-1 Glass
Lunch	Vegetable-1 Katori
	Boiled Soft Khichri-1 Katori
	Curd-1/2 Katori
Evening	Milk-1 Glass
	Toast-2 Slices
Dinner	Daal-1 Katori
	Vegetable Soup-1 Bowl
	Meat curry-1 Katori
	Paratha-1 no
	Moong Salad-1 Plate
Bed Time	Milk with Ice Cream-1/2 Katori

Diet for Child (3-4 Yrs)

Early Morning	Mango Milk Shake-1 Glass
Break Fast	Hot Buttered Toast-2 Slice
	Egg-1no
Mid Morning	Sugar Cane juice-1 Glass
Lunch	Rajmah Curry-1 K atori
	Rice-1 Katori
	Kadhi-1 Katori

	Carrot Salad-1 Plate
	Sahi Paneer-1 Katori
Evening	Banana Shake-1 Glass
Dinner	Palak Paneer Curry-1 Katori
	Dry Mix Sabji-1 Katori
	Parathas-2 nos.
	Salad-1 Plate
Bed Time	Kheer-1/2 Katori

Diet for Child (5-6 Yrs)

Early Morning	Milk-1 Glass
Break Fast	Cheese Toast-2 Slices
Mid Morning	Stuffed Idlee-1no
Lunch	Channa Curry-1 Katori
	Boiled Rice-1 Katori
	Carrot and Cucumber Salad-1 Plate
	Mint Raita-1 Katori
Evening	Banana Shake-1 Glass
	Bread Roll with Sprouts-1 katori
Dinner	Potato and Paneer Curry-1 Katori
	Dry Tinda-1 Katori
	Roti-2 nos.
	Salad-1 Plate
BT	Cabbage Kheer-1/2 Katori

Diet for School Child

School child refers to children from the age of 8 years to 12 years. During the school years the rate of growth slow down. Growth continues at steady pace. School years are known as by an improvement of the functioning of most tissues and organs system. It is important that growth and development of muscles and bones takes place. The influences of nutrients play vital role for growth and development. Good nutrition need good development. Providing sufficient nutrients to support growth and development, the vigorous activity of school years makes demand on the body. Physical activity needs energy. The child who had vigorous physical activity obviously need more energy. Heavy activity means more perspiration and losses of water and minerals like Sodium and Potassium. Therefore satisfactory dietary patterns and food habits help to ensure healthy child.

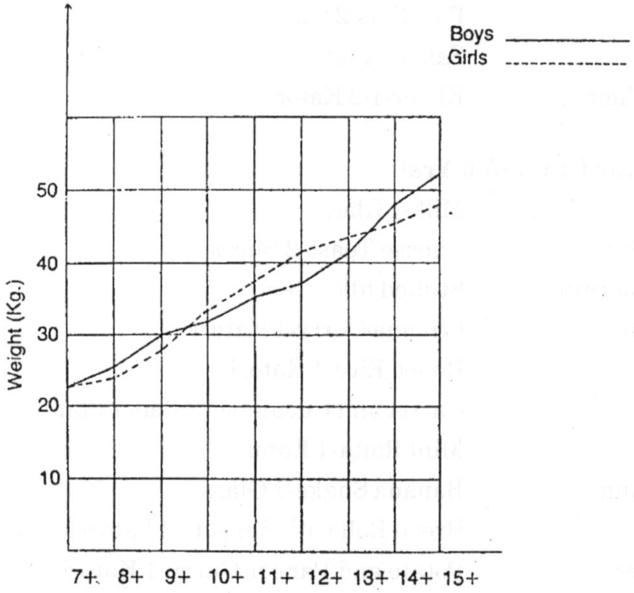

Sex differences in growth during the school years.

Recommended Dietary Allowances

Nutrients	*RDI* *7-9 years*	*Age group* *10-12 years*
Energy	1950	2190
Protein	41	54
Calcium	400	600
Iron	26	34
Vitamin A	600	600
Thiamine	2400	2400
Riboflavin	1.0	1.1
Niacin	1.2	1.3
Vitamin B	0.2	1.0

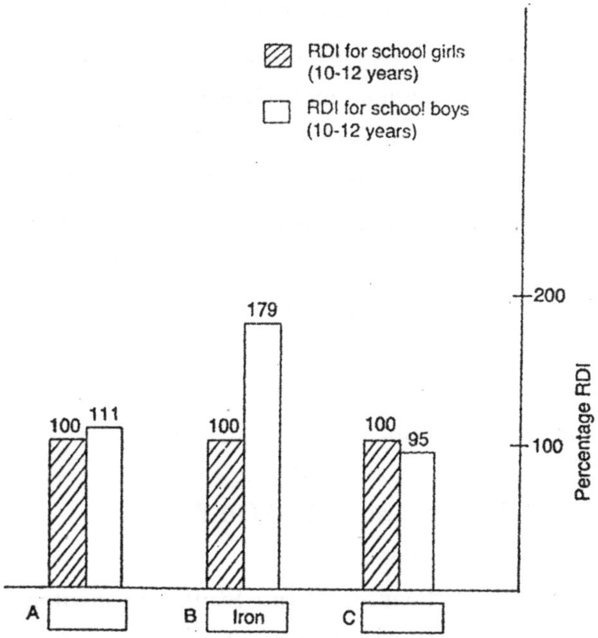

Comparison between RDI for school girls and boys (10-12 yrs.)

Recommended Allowances

Protein	-	60 gms
Calcium	-	400 gms
Calories	-	2000
Vitamin A	-	2400

Diet for Adolescent Individual (08 Yrs)

Early Morning	Milk with Maltova-1 Glass
Break Fast	Mango Shake-1 Glass
	Paneer Sandwitch-2 Slices
	Guava-1no.
Lunch	Daal-1 Katori
	Boiled Rice-1 Plate
	Veg. Pulao-1 Katori

	Kheera Salad-1 Plate
	Curd-1K/Raita-1 Katori
	Paneer matar-1 Katori
Evening	Umpa-1 Katori
Dinner	Daal-1 Katori
	Stuffed Tinda-1 Katori
	Roti-2 no
	Salad-1 Plate
	Raita-1 Katori
	Mutton Kabab-1 Stick
Bed time	Milk Custard thin-1 Glass

Diet for Adolescent Individual (10 Yrs)

Break Fast	Milk-1 Glass
	Peas and Potato Stuffed Sandwitch-2 Slices
Mid day	Paneer Paratha-2 nos.
	Peach-1 no.
Lunch	Sambhar-1 Katori
	Boiled Rice-1 Plate
	Kheera Salad-1 Plate
	Curd-1 Katori
Evening	Cold Coffee-1 Cup
	Poha-1 Plate
Dinner	Urad whole Daal-1 Katori
	Stuffed Capsicum-1 Katori
	Roti-2 nos.
	Salad-1 Plate
Bed Time	Fruit Custard-1 Katori

Diet for Adolescent Individual (11 Yrs)

Break Fast	Paneer Stuffed Parathas-2 nos.
	Green Chutney-1/2 Katori

	Milk-1 Glass
Mid Day	Banana-1 no
	Radish Stuffed Roti-1 no
	Egg Bhujia-1 Katori
Lunch	Moong Daal Khichri-1 Katori
	Roti-1 no
	Curd Salad-1 Plate
	Chicken Grilled-1 Pc
Evening	Peanut with Murmura-1 Katori
	Apple-1 no
	Fruit juice-1 Glass
Dinner	Daal-1 Katori
	Potato Gazar Sabji-1 Katori
	Rice/Roti
	Curd-1 Katori
Bed Time	Sweet Phirni-1 Katori

Diet for Adolescent Individual (12 Yrs)

Break Fast	Thin Lassi-1 Glass
	Missi Roti-2
	Green chutney-1/2 Katori
Mid Day	Missi Roti-2 nos.
	Radish Bhujia-1 Katori
Lunch	Spinach Moong Daal-1 Katori
	Roti-2
	Carrot Salad-1 Plate
Evening	Tea-1 Cup
	Peanut with Murmura-1 Katori
	Guava-1no
Dinner	Daal with Vegetable-1 Katori
	Potato Sabji-1 Katori

	Rice/Roti
Bed Time	Sweet Curd-1 Katori

Diet for Adolescents

Teenagers undergo rapid growth. Therefore it is necessary to take care of their nutrition and their growth does not become stunted. A poor diet is often inadequate both in calories and calcium. A deficient supply of calcium may also lead to reduction in food intake and further stunt the growth. There is an adequate supply of calories the deficiency of calcium will result in an uneven body development.

Malnutrition at this stage can impair body function, working ability, physical growth and skeletal development.

The period of adolescent is one of considerable stress in terus of physical growth, hormonal changes and emotional strain. Food requirements, i.e. Protein, Calcium and Iron are increased. The increased need for protein is conditioned by "spurt" in growth in when occurs at puberty. In boys height gin about 20cm and weight gin about 18 kg. In girls it is a bit less.

Calcium requirement at this age is high and Iron requirement for girls 30-35 mg and for boys 20-25 mgs.

Recommended Dietary Allowances

Nutrients	*RDI* *10-12 Yrs (Boys)*	*Age group* *10-12 Yrs (Girls)*
Energy	2190	1970
Protein	54	57
Calcium	600	600
Iron	34	19
Vitamin-A	3000	3000
Thiamine	1.1	1.0
Riboflavin	1.3	1.2
Niacin	13	15
Vitamin-E	40	40
Folic Acid	70	70

Recommended Allowances

Protein	-	60 gm.
Calcium	-	0.5-1.0 gm.
Calories	-	3000 gm.
Vitamin A	-	3000 mg.

Diet for Adolescent Individual (14 Yrs)

Break Fast	Porridge-1 Bowl
	Boiled Egg-1 no
Mid Morning	Daal-1 Katori
	Palak Parathas-1 no
	Orange-1 no
Lunch	Kadhi-1 Katori
	Stuffed Brinjal-1 Katori
	Boiled Rice-1 Katori
	Salads-1 Katori
Evening	Cold Coffee-1 Cup
	Vegetable Cutlet-2 nos.
Dinner	Pea and Keema Curry-1 Katori
	Cauliflower Potato Dry-1 Katori
	Rash wali Sabji-1 Katori
	Roti-2
Bed Time	Fruits Custard-1 Katori

Diet for Adolescent Individual (15 Yrs)

Break Fast	Corn Flakes-1 Katori
	Apple-1 no
Mid Morning	Stuffed Daal Parathas-1 no
	Green chutney-1 Tsp
	Orange-1 no
Lunch	Raita-1 Katori
	Stuffed Karela-1 Katori
	Boiled Rice-1 Plate
	Veg Polao-1 Katori
	Salads-1 Plate

	Grilled Paneer-1 Plate
Evening	Keema Cutlet-2 nos.
	Mango Shake-1 Glass
Dinner	Pea Mutton Masala-1 Katori
	Dry Brinjal-1 Katori
	Rash wali Sabji-1 Katori
	Roti-2 nos
Bed Time	Ice Cream-1 scoop

Diet for Adolescent Individual (17 Yrs)

Break fast	Veg. Upma-1 Katori
	Milk-1 Glass
Mid Day	Apple-1 no
	Orange-1 no
Lunch	Paneer Pulao-1 Katori
	Salads-1 Plate
	Raita-1 Katori
	Tinda Dry Sabji-1 Katori
Evening	Banana-1 no
	Paneer Tikki-1/2 Plate
Dinner	Mushroom Sabji-1 Bowl
	Mutton Kabab-1 Stick
	Gobhi Mussalam-1/2 Plate
	Mint/Carrot Raita-1 Katori
	Roti-2 nos.
Bed Time	Milk-1 Glass

Diet for Adolescent Individual (18 Yrs)

Break Fast	French Toast-2 Slices
	Milk-1 Glass
	Apple-1 no
Lunch	Channas-1 Katori
	Methi Aloo-1 Katori
	Salads-1 Plate
	Poori-3 nos.

Evening	Banana Milk Shake-1 Glass
	Capsicum Pizza-1/2 Plate
Dinner	Cream Mushroom Soup-1 Bowl
	Keema Kofta Curry-1 Katori
	Gobhi Mussalam-1/2 Plate
	Carrot Raita-1 Katori
	Tandoori Roti-2 nos.
Bed Time	Fruit with Cream-1 Katori

Diet for Adults

While Planning diets for adulthood kindly consider on their specific occupation, which varying is calorie requirements. Requirements of calorie for adult men and women will depend on various type of activity. Men need mare than women because of their height, weight and the type of occupation. Diets for adults should have sufficient amounts of all the essential nutrients. The meal can be increased by variety of food. Occupations of the adults can generally be classified as follows :

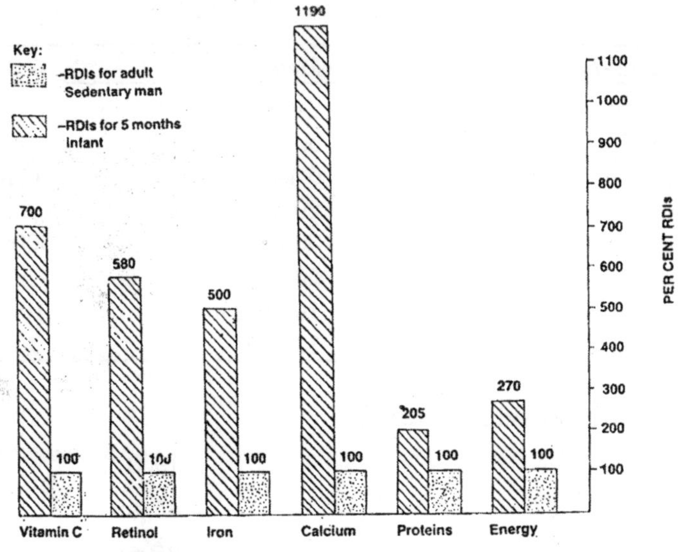

Foods to Emphasize during Pregnancy.

In addition to physical activity and to the type and nature of occupational activities, the energy requirement of individuals also depends on factors such as body size and composition, age, sex and climate.

Light Work *Sedentary Worker*		*Moderately Active* *Active Worker*		*Very Active* *Heavy Worker*	
Men 2400kcal	women 1900kcal	Men 2800kcal	Women 2200kacl	Men 3900kcal	Women 3000kcal
Officeworker ,lawers, doctor, accountants, teacher, architects	Officeworker ,lawers, doctor, accountants, teacher, architects	Industry worker, construction worker,farm worker	Housewife, Servent, Store worker,	Agricultural worker, labourer, soldier, mines worker,steel worker	Farm worker, Dancer, athletes,

Recommended Dietary Allowances

Nutrients	*Men*	*Women*
Energy	2400	1900
Protein	55	45
Calcium	0.4-0.5	0.4-0.5
Iron	20 mg	30 mg
Vitamin-A	3000 mg	3000mg
Ascarbic Acid	50 mg	50 mg
Folic Acid	100 mg.	100 mg
Riboflavin	1.3-2.2	1.0-1.7

Recommended Allowances

Calories	-	1900
Protein	-	45 gm
Iron	-	35 gm
Vitamin-C	-	50 mg

Diet for Adults (Male and Female)
1st Phase Plan

Early Morning	Tea-1Cup
Break fast	Broken Wheat Porridge-1 Bowl
	Poached Egg-1 no
	Toast with Butter-2 Slices
	Apple-1 no
Mid Day	Coffee-1 Cup
	Biscuit-2 nos.
Lunch	Lentil Daal-1 Katori
	Palak Saag-1 Katpori
	Salad-1 Plate
	Roti-2 nos.
	Fruit Custard-1 Katori
Evening	Vegetable Upma-1 Plate
	Tea-1 Cup
Dinner	Lauki Kofta Curry-1 Katrori
	Potato Cauliflower dry Sabji-1 Katori
	Bhoondi Raita-1 Katori
	Carrot Greated Salad-1 Plate
	Roti/Rice
Bed Time	Milk-1 Glass

Diet for Adulthood (Male and Female)
2nd Phase Plan

Early Morning	Tea-1 Cup
Break Fast	Light Daal Khichri-1 Katori
	Boiled Egg-1 no
	Tea-1 Cup
Mid Day	Papaya-1 Plate
Lunch	Daal Palak-1 Katori

	Salad-1 Plate
	Roti-2 nos.
	Rice-1 Katori
	Fish/Chicken-1 Katori
Evening	Idlee with chutney -1 Plate
	Tea-1 Cup
Dinner	Soup-1 Bowl
	Carrot Greated Salad-1 Plate
	Roti/Rice
	Urad Daal-1 Katori
	dry Sabji-1 Katori
Bed Time	Kheer-1 Katori

Diet for Pregnancy

Pregnancy is a period of great physiological as well as psychological stress for the women. She has to maintain her health at optimum level to prepare for delivery and lactation,

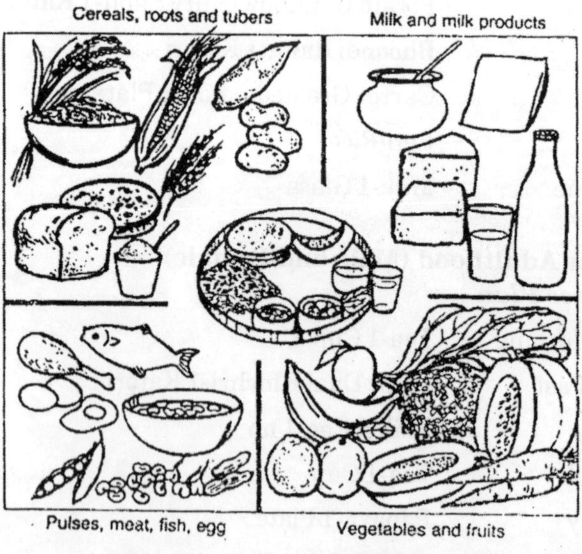

Nutrients needs of infants as compared to those of an adult man.

and provide good nutrition for the development of the fetus. Due to fetus grows rapidly, the nutritional needs are increased for building materials for the formation of new tissues. So diet for the pregnant woman must provide for the additional requirements.

Nutritional deficiency increased chances of infection owing to a decrease in normal body function. So qualitative and quantitative changes in the diet are essential during pregnancy. Poor food intake during pregnancy is not of poverty. Often poor woman is anemic to begin with thus gets aggravated during pregnancy. So times hemoglobin could be much less than 10 per cent. In that case the anemia needs to be corrected.

The pregnant woman is not able to eat much at a time therefore must space between the meals must include drinks, i.e., buttermilk, milk, lemon juice, simple snacks between meals.

Under nutrition during pregnancy is also found in the high income groups.

The common saying that "A pregnant woman must eat for two".

Recommended Dietary Allowances

Nutrients	*RDI*
Calories	Normal (1900) + 300
Protein	Normal (45) + 10
Calcium	Normal (0.4) + 1.0
Iron	30
Vitamin-A	6000
Thiamine	2.2
Riboflavin	1.6
Ascorbic Acid	80
Folic Acid	2.5
Vitamin-D	1.2

Diet during Pregnancy

Early Morning Coffee-1 Cup

Break fast Tea-1 Cup

	Cheese Sandwitch-2 Slices
Lunch	Fruit Custard-1 Katori
	Mutton Curry-1 Katori
	Mix Dry Sabji-1 Katori
	Ghia Raita-1 Katori
	Rice/Roti
	Salad-1 Plate
Evening	Banana-2 nos.
	Bhel-1 Katori
Dinner	Paneer Sahi wali-1 Katori
	Urad Daal-1 Katori
	Roti-2 nos.
	Raita-1 Katori
Bed time	Fruit Custard-1 Katori

Diet during Pregnancy

BreakFast	Tea-1 Cup
	Palak Besan Parathas-1 no
Mid Morning	Guava-1 no
	Biscuit-2 nos.
	Nimbu Pani-1 Glass
Lunch	Channa Curry-1 Katori
	Stuffed Tinda-1 Katori
	Pudina Raita-1 Katori
	Rice/Roti
	Salad-1 Plate
Evening	Banana Shake-1 Glass
	Poha-1 Plate
Dinner	Paneer Matar Curry-1 Katori
	Mix Daal-1 Katori
	Roti/Rice
Bed Time	Fruit Custard-1 Katori

Diet for Lactation

During lactation increase in the nutrients are depend on the quality of milk secreted. The production capacity which is an individual physiologic characteristic influenced by the environment. Emotional factors also diminish the secretion of milk depends on adequate diet. Deficiencies in the food can decrease the secretion of milk and its quality Dietary needs of a lactating mother are even greater than that of a pregnant woman to person. The mother secretes about ½ liter of milk per day in the first meal which increases up to about 1 liter. The lactating mother needs approximate about 400 calories additive. The diet pattern during pregnancy, but it is advisable to increase the intake of foods like milk and calories. Decrease of emotional disturbance are good for lactation.

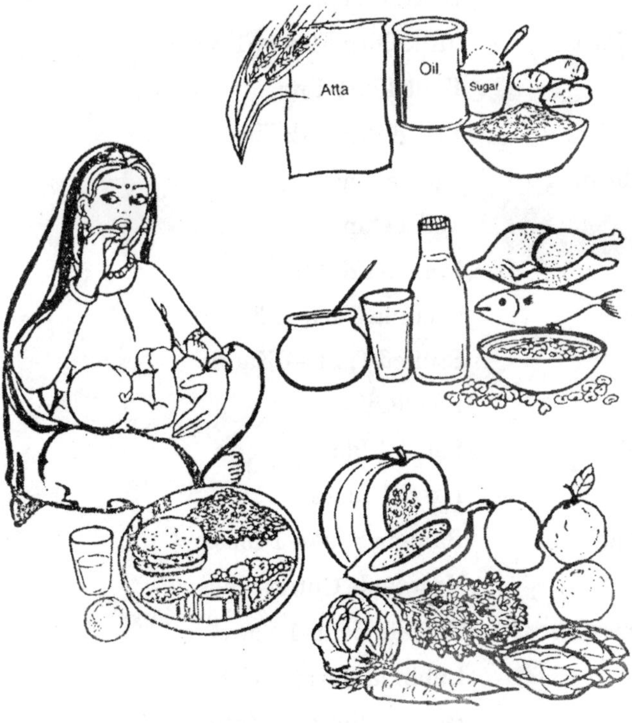

Foods to essential during Lactation.

Recommended Dietary Allowances

Nutrients	*RDI*
Calories	Normal (1900) + 700
Protein	Normal (45) + 20
Calcium	0.4 + 1.0
Iron	30
Vitamin-A	5750
Thiamine	1.5
Riboflavin	1.4
Ascorbic Acid	30
Folic Acid	25
Vitamin B_{12}	1+0.2

Diet during Lactation

Early Morning	Milk-1 Glass
	Biscuit-3 nos.
BreakFast	Milk Corn Flakes-1 Bowl
	Boiled Egg-1 no
	Bread Butter-2 Slice
Mid Morning	Guava-1 no
	Tea-1 Cup
	Phirni-1 Katori
Lunch	Channa Curry-1 Katori
	Stuffed Tinda-1 Katori
	Rice/Roti
	Salad-1 Plate
	Lassi-1 Glass
Evening	Banana Shake-1 Glass
	Vegetable Cutlet-2 nos.
Dinner	Tomato Soup-1 Bowl
	Lubhiya Curry-1 Katori
	Brinjal Bharta-1 Katori
	Potato Raita-1 Katori

	Roti/Rice
Bed Time	Milk-1 Glass

Diet during Lactation

Early Morning	Coffee- 1 C
Break Fast	Milk with Walnut-1 Bowl
	Egg Sandwitch-2 Slices
Mid day	Tea-1 Cup
	Carrot Kheer-1 Katori
Lunch	Chicken Curry-1 Katori
	Stuffed Parmal-1 Katori
	Rice/Roti
	Sprouts Salad-1 Plate
Evening	Walnut Milk Shake-1 Glass
	Toast-2 Slices
Dinner	Ghia Soup-1 Bowl
	Black Channa Curry-1 Katori
	Brinjal Aloo Sabji-1 Katori
	Curd Raita-1 Katori
	Roti/Rice
	Roasted Chicken-1 Pcs
Bed Time	Milk Banana Shake-1 Glass

16
Food Adulteration

For good health we must take good food; it connotes not only a nutritionally balanced diet but also wholesome and safe food. The consumer in general not a producer himself, depends upon the market and is blissfully ignorant of the insidious hazards of consuming adultrated foods. Foods may be adulterated either intentionally or accidentally at all stages from production to retail. The additives affect the food in colour, shape, size and appearance in such a way that it becomes difficult for an average buyer to detect adulteration at first sight. In each case the quality of food is deliberately lowered in order to derive maximum profit from sale. A consumer tends to be guided mostly by the price, visual appeal and the claims made by the advertisements.

What is Quality ?

Quality can be defined as "that make a thing what it is, nature, characteristics, kind, property, status, grade of goodness and excellence"

The parameter of the quality are the grades, standards and specifications laid down by the government or expert bodies constitutes for the purpose. An established system of quality control assures uniformity accepted standard and thereby ensures that each foodstuffs is what its purpose to be and what its label claim to be. It is said that quality is never an accident, it is always the results of intelligent effort. There must be a will to produce superior articles.

The standard of the food set by the government. The chemical composition of different articles of food have been worked out and legal standards of purity have been prescribed. These standards constitute the bais of assess ment of purity of the food products. Articles of food are chemically analysised by food chemists in the laboratory and are measured against these yard sticks to ascertain if they satisfy the requirements laid down in this regard. They are adulterated if they do not measure upto the prescribed standard.

A variety of food and other items are purchased in all homes. A lot of one's hard earned money is spent on food alone. Have you cooked at the wheat that has been procured for your family?

Is it Clean?

Is the wheat mixed with similar cooking mud balls and some things ?

Are all the grains healthy or some shrunken grains are also present in the wheat purchased ?

Is the Wheat Worm-infested?

You must be knowledgeable enough to distinguish between good quality and inferior quality foods. Make that you are not being cheated. It will also ensure that you get your money's worth.

After reading this chapter you will be able to :

- Define and explain the meaning of adulteration.
- Differentiate 'between adulterant and adulteration.
- Enumerate factors under which the food is considered adultered according to the Prevention of Food adulteration Act (PFA).
- Enlist some of the adulterate present in commonly used foods.
- Enumerate hazards due to commonly present adulterate.

- Discuss steps taken for protection against adulteration.
- Describe simple tests of defection of the adulterant present in the food.
- Enumerate the measures to safeguard against food adulteration.
- Appreciate that the standard marks safeguard the consumer against food adulteration.

Definition and Meaning of Adulteration

The food is considered adultered in the following instances :

(a) Addition of cheap and inferior substances lesser the quality of foods purchased. For example—Water in milk, vanaspati in pure ghee.

(b) Removal of valuable component also lowers and deteriorates the quality of food. For example—Remove cream from milk.

(c) Addition of harmful substances to good food endangers health. For example—Metanil yellow used in burfi, laddu, haldi.

What is Adulteration ?

The way in which the quality of food is lowered is called adulteration. It can be defined as "lowering the quality of food by adding cheap/inferior substances to of or by removing an important part of it or by presence of harmful substances in the food.

Food adulteration can be incidental or intentional. Intentional adulteration of food is done to make more profit while the incidental adulteration is due to negligence, i.e., some harmful substances getting mixed with food accidentally.

What is an Adulterant ?

An Adulterant can be defined as 'any cheap outside item which looks the same as the original item which looks the same as the original food stuff, which mixed very well with it and is not very easy to detect'. These are : stone, chips, mud balls, grit, bark, twigs and parts of plant, similar seeds, starch, sugar, powdered seeds, san dust.

When is the Food Adultered ?

Prevention of Food Adulteration Act 1954 (PFA) describes the conditions under which the food considered adultered. The act came into force on 1st June, 1955. The rules since then have been amended in 1968 and 1973 to safeguard the consumers. Food is considered adulterated :

(a) When the nature, substance and quality differ from what it ought to be.

(b) If it contains injurious ingredients.

(c) If it contains cheaper/inferior substances.

(d) If any constituent has been removed/abstracted partially or wholly from it.

(e) If it is infested with insects/worms etc.

(f) If it is prepared, packed and stored under unsanitary conditions.

(g) If it is obtained from sick/diseased animal.

(h) If it contains poisonous ingredients that are injurious to health.

(i) If it contains unpermitted colour. Food is also considered adulterated if it contains excessive amounts of the permitted colours.

(j) If it contains prohibited preservatives. Food is also considered adulterated if it contains excessive amounts of the permitted preservatives.

(k) If it contains chemically react with the food and makes it poisonous and injurious to health.

(l) If it does not satisfy the prescribed standards laid down by authorities.

Commonly Used Foods and the Adulterants Present. You will now study about the various adulterants present in the foods commonly used is most households.

Cereals : Stones, grit, mud balls are often present in wheat, rice and bajra. Dry things and stems are also mixed with the cereals to increase the weight.

Pulses : Whole daals often have similar stones and metanil yellow also used to enhance the colour.

Sugar, Honey and Jaggery : May have chalk powder and fine chips as the adulterant present in it. Thick syrup add in honey.

Ghee and Oil : Vanaspati add in pure ghee to make more profits. Cheaper oil mix oil mustard oil.

Milk : Addition of water and removal of cream from milk lower the quality of milk.

Tea and Coffee : Used and colored tea leaves are the common adulterants responsible for lowing the quality and grade of tea. Coffee is adulterated with chicory beans powder.

Salt and Spices : Salt may be mixed with chalk powder, dirt and stones. Spice powders are often adulterated with excessive amounts of sand, straw, sawdust or cow dung.

Health Hazards of Common Adulterants

Adulterants	*Food Adulterated*	*Hazards*
Stone, chips, mud Balls, grit and sawdust	Cereals, pulses, jaggery and spices	Stomach upset stones can damage teeth and intestine.
Kesari Dal	Channa dal, Arhar dal, besan, and moong dal powder	Consumption of kesari dal causes paralysis of lower limbs
Metanil Yellow	Enhance the colour of Dal, besan haldi etc.	They crippling disease is called lathyrilsm and mainly attacks boys and men between the ages of 5-45 yrs.

Talcum powder Asbestos powder	Pulses are mixed with talcum and asbestos powder	
Argemine oil	Mustard oil help Adultered with cheap oil	Causing stomach trouble, liver and kidney damage
Rhodamine B	Red chillies	Stomach upset, kidney stone and stomach cancer
Mineral oil	Edible oil	Partial and total blindness and hazards of heart. Trouble in liver, kidney and spleen. It cannot absorb by body

Detection of Adulterant Present in Foods

Cereals. Should be picked and cleaned before cooking them. The stones, twigs and other plants parts can be seen and picked. Washing of the cereals grains enables one to remove the mud and dirt.

Pulses. Visual check of pulses will enable one to separate the kesari daal from the arhar and chana dals. Put some dal in a test tube; Add water and shake. Add dilute HCI (Hydrochloric Acid) and shake. Presence of magenta red colour shows that the dal is adultered with metanil yellow.

Milk and Milk Products. Addition of water and starch, removal cream lower the quality of milk. Transfer milk from one glass to another, milky appearance of the empty glass suggests that the milk is pure. The lactometer test can be done in the laboratory to find out the specific gravity/density of milk. The specific gravity of pure milk is 1.030-1.034. Starch used in khoya, burfi etc.

Tea and Coffee. Iron filing in tea leaves can easily be defected with the help of a magnet. Tamarind seeds also present in coffee. Put some amount of potassium hydroxide solution on top. Emergence of brown colour and coffee particles confirms adulteration.

Salt. Dissolve the sample of salt in a beaker, dirt settle at the base and salt dissolve in water.

Black Pepper. It looks like similar to papaya seeds at casual glance. Papaya seeds have rough surface as black pepper. Papaya seeds are lighter than black pepper.

Protection Against Food Adulteration

Adulteration of commonly used foods in increasing at an alarming pace. The cost of food is forever increasing and the unscrupulous traders are indulging in malpractices to increase their profit margin. You should safeguard yourself from the menace of adulteration in the following ways :

1. Buy from reliable shops only. If you buy from a shop that has reputation and large sales turnover, you will be able to get fresh and good quality stocks.
2. Buy standard and reliable brands of foods for they will be good quality. Look for the standard marks for getting the full value of your money. Standard marks safeguard against food.

Standard Marks of Foods

The Bureau of Indian Standard (BIS) stands guarantee for the quality of products bearing ISI mark. Indian Standards Institution mark ensures that : (a) The quality of foods particularly those affecting health and safety of consumers is superb. (b) The mass produced and mass consumed products confirm to the required standards of quality, safety and durability.

There is a wide range of consumer goods that carry the ISI mark. As a quality conscious consumer you must look for this mark before purchasing anything. A list of the commodities bearing mark is given below :

Air conditioner, Helmets, Immersion heater, Ceiling fan, Ink pen, Stone, Gas stove, Aluminum vessels, Cooking range,

Safety match, Refrigeration, Door closers, Shaving blades, Napthalene balls, Liquid toilet soap, Detergent powder, Handloom cotton, Bed sheets, Sewing thread, Vanaspati, Baby foods, Biscuits, Coffee powder, Edible, common salt, Chewing gum.

Agmark determines the quality and purity of the agricultural products. The word AGMARK is a derivative of agricultural marketing. The quality of the product is assessed on the basis of production, varies size, shape, weight, colour, moisture, fat content and other relevant physical and chemical characteristics. Agmark products are available in grocery stones, super bazaars and departmental stores. Some of the products bearing Agmark are as follows :

Rice, Mustard oil, Wheat, Pure ghee, Pulses, Butter, Gram flour, Honey, Mangoes, Spices, Grapes, Curry powder, Citrus fruits, Black pepper powder, Coconut oil, Eggs, Tea, etc.

Look for "Agmark" symbol on the products you purchase next time and be sure about the purity of the product and the quality of your decision.

I. **PFA.** Prevention of Food Adulteration Act 1954 controls that the foods and their products are not adulterated.

II. **FPO.** Stands for Fruit Products Order and was founded by the government of India in 1946 under the defense of India rules. FPO lays down minimum standards relating to the quality of various fruits and vegetables products. The order specifies the standard of sanitation and hygiene to be followed in the factories, besides giving directions regarding packing, marking, and labeling. If the manufacturer does not confirm to these regulations, he is liable to be punished under the provision of the law.

The Food Bearing Marks are

Jam, Baked Beans, Syrups, Jellies, Sardines, Pickles, Marmalade, Soap, Chutnies, Ketchup, Squashes.

III. Do not buy loose food stuffs wherever sealed packets and tins are available. It is easier to adulterate loose food materials than temper with the packet stuff.

IV. Study the label and the standard mark before purchasing the food stuff. A good label provides the consumer with the following information :

(i) Name of the food stuffs.

(ii) Ingredients contained.

(iii) Date of manufacturing and date of expiry.

(iv) Name, place and address of manufacturer.

(v) Net contents and cast excluding local taxes.

(vi) Instructions for storage and use.

(vii) Standard mark for quality product.

V. Be quality conscious and sure that you are not being cheated by adulteration. In case you suspect the shopkeeper on the manufacturer of adulating the food stuff do notify to the concerned authorities for proper action. Public health laboratories test and analyze adulterated food stuff. These laboratories work under the guidance of central food laboratories. The seller and manufacturer if found guilty can even get life imprisonment. These laboratories are situated at Collate, Pine, My sore and Ghazi bad.

Besides government agencies already mentioned, certain voluntary agencies also contribute to check the menace of adulteration. These are :

(a) Quality control laboratories of food company's, e.g., canning industry.

(b) Quality control laboratories of consumer organizations, e.g., super bazaar.

(c) Private testing laboratories.

Besides the standard marks studies so far, you may have also heard of eco-mark. It is put on products that are environment friendly or eco-friendly. It ensures that the product is biogradable and will not pollute the environment.

Have you seen wool mark ? When you see this wool mark on woolen cloth, you can be sure of its quality and purity.

Possible Health Hazards of Hawker's School Snacks

Name of the Snacks	*Adulterates*	*Health Hazards*
Aam Papad	Dust, insect excreta	Nausea, vomiting
Ice candy	Metanil yellow	Diarrhoea, Abdominal pain
Karachi Halwa males, cancer	Metanil yellow	Degerration of tests in
Rasgulla	Poisonous colour	Lesions in ritual organ lungs, eyes
Sugar coated saunf		Abnormalities in bone.
Coconut churan	Sawdust	S mental retardation stomach irritation.
Supari	Melachite green Auramine dirt	Brain damage
Toffee	Soap stone	Stomach cancer
Moong Dal Ground nut	Metanil yellow	Degeneration of testes Fungus and fungal toxin Liver damage

Health Hazards due to Metal Contamination

Metal are toxic when present beyond a small concentration. In the beginning they combine with proteins and this neutralizes the poisioning effect. When the concentration increases rapidly very quick onset of symptoms such as vomiting, nausea, and pain in the stomach arises.

1. Arsenic—Arsenic pesticides are the main sources of arsenic contaminants.Arsenic in the form of salts is easily absorbed in the gastro intestinal tract. Apples are sprayed over with lead arsenate which is harmful for human beings.Arsenic if taken in concentrated form

is very harmful, producing dazziness, chills, cramps, paralysis and death.

2. Lead—It present in food stuffs like shellfish, herbs, edible gelatin, peptin, food colouring, tea, baking powder, custard and peaches. Llead brings changes in kidney and arteries thus shortening life.

   Exposure to lead :

   - Contact with packing equipments.
   - Lead pipes through drinking water is obtained.
   - Use of turmeric powder in which lead chromate present.
   - Use of citric acid and synthetic dyes.
   - Spraying and dusting of fruits and vegetables.
   - Use of lead containing pesticides such as lead arsenate.

3. Tin—A variety of containers made of tin plate are also used for string oils, fats, beverages, biscuits, and all types of processed foods. Poisioning foods causes severe headache, vomiting, photophobia, abdominal pain, dehydration and retention of urine.

Tin poisoning may result :

- When canned food is acidic.
- When the food is acidic.
- When the food contains nitrates and oxalates.
- When food contains copper and sulphur.
- When food left moist.

4. Copper—Copper causes diarrhea, abdominal pain, vomiting, construction in the throat, astringent taste with thirst.

5. Aluminium—Sweets and meat were always covered with siver foils which cause undesirable reactions in digestive tract, interfering with the normal functions.

6. Xadmium—Which is a silvery soft white metal is used for plating utensils and electric cookers. It dissolve

in food and can be harmful to health after ingestion of food.

Health Hazards due to Bacterial and Fungal Contamination

Bacteria and fungal palys vital role in public health. Poor methods of cultivation, harvest, processing, transportation, storage, distribution and preparation for consumption, create favourable conditions for foood contamination. Food which are easily contaminated are milk, milk products, meat and meat products, poultry, egg, fish, raw vegetables, fruits and cereals.

Sign of bacterial and fungal contaminations :

- Change in appearance, texture, odour, flavour of food.
- Loose, fuzzy, velvety growth of food.
- Surface of food looks whity, slimmy and liquid.

Health Hazards due to Pests and Pesticides

Pest such as rodents and insects cause contamination on food. Once they get into food,they consume a lot of it. They leave filth, bodily secretions, insect, fragments and rodent hairs as well as disease bearing and spoilage micro organism.

1. *Rodent.* It includes rats and mice. A single rat voids 10.000 dropping and 4 liters of urine annually, and 5 lakhs of hairs. The kidney of these rodents have an organism causes disease of the liver, it transmitted to man through food and water. Rats causes 35 diseases.
2. *Insects.* Such as beetles, weevils, borers, make short work of stored food like cereals, pulses and flours. They eat up the whole grains and in this process uric acid and an offensive odour and taste develop in the food.
3. *Pesticides.* Organic pesticides like DDT, BHC, malthin, pyrethrum are used but these leave behind on the food as a residue, the unchanged chemicals or their derivatives. These are toxic depending on the nature

of potential killers, the maximum concentration of pesticide residue that is permitted in or on food is laid down by the P.H.A. Acute poisioning by DDT are rare but continued consumption of these may lead to chronic health problems.

Health Hazards due to Packing

The most common packing material in the food industry is PVC and PE. This plastic material is contaminated with noxious thermal break down products of the plastics welding, heat sealing or sterilizing pickles containing fats and acids may react with the components of plastic packaging and prove a health hazards.

A Citizen's Duty

1. it is the duty of every citizen to assist in curbing the menace of adulteration. Do not over look instances of adulteration. Take an active interest in exposing and condemning them.
2. be active in giving information about specific instances of adulteration.
3. give lawful assistance to food inspectors in drawing of samples of adulterated articles.
4. be ready to act as a witness and to give evidence in court in such cases.
5. offer full cooperation and help in drives against adulterated foods.
6. you should not purchase cheap adulterated foods.
7. always prefer to purchase AG marks or ISI marks tins.
8. remember the slogan "adulteration is a menace to health".

Malpractices of Food Dealers

When demand is more than supply dealer get chance to indulge in malpractices. These in turn affect the economic situation and the health of the consumer. Dealers may try to cheat the consumer by following means :

1. adulteration.
2. defective weight and measures.
3. inadequate labeling.
4. false advertisement.

The problems of the customers is how, when and what quality of goods is to be bought so as to get the best value for the money. To use his money wisely, a consumer need to be, fully informed about prices which may vary from one market to another. The best course is to take advantage of the large number of cooperative stores in Indian cities. The choice of which store to buy from is also influenced by the type of services it offers to consumers display, coutesy, home delivery and credit facilities.

17
Nutrients and its Deficiency Symptoms

Arsenic

Although most commonly known for its toxic properties, arsenic (As) has been shown to have beneficial actions when fed in very small amounts to laboratory animals. Numerous studies with rats, hamsters, minipigs, goats, and chicks have provided circumstantial evidence suggesting that arsenic is essential, but its physiological role has not been clearly defined. However, there is evidence that arsenic intake affects taurine and polyamine concentrations in plasma and tissues.

Deficiencies. The most impressive reported sign of arsenic deficiency is decreased growth of goats, impaired success of the first service and conception rates, greater absorption of fetuses during pregnancy, and higher mortality rate during the second lactation. There is often sudden death, and the mitochondria of the cardiac muscle showed ultra structural changes in deficient goats. The most consistent signs of arsenic deprivation in rodents are decreased growth, higher death rate of young, rougher and yellowish hair coats (in white rats), elevated erythrocytes osmotic fragility, elevated spleen iron and splenomegaly. However, the severity and variation of these deficiency signs depend upon several dietary factors including the zinc, arginine, choline, methionine and guanidoacetic acid content. These substances are interrelated because they are effectors of methionine metabolism. Arsenic-deprived chicks drank and excreted more water, exhibited slower growth, usually had leg abnormalities, and arginine-supplemented deficient chicks had elevated hepatic zinc levels but depressed content of arsenic, iron and manganese in this tissue. Arsenic may be important under certain circumstances in humans. For example, arsenic, independent of omega-3 fatty acids, increases bleeding time. This implies that it may be a plausible candidate for the unknown factor in fish responsible for increased bleeding time. In addition, a recent human study suggested that arsenic homeostasis is altered by hemodialysis, and that low serum arsenic is correlated with central nervous system disorders, vascular disease, and "possibly" cancer.

Diet recommendations. It is inappropriate at present to give dietary recommendations for arsenic for humans because of questions of its essentiality. Based on animal studies, however, amounts of arsenic in the diet that lead to signs of arsenic deficiency can be extrapolated to humans. The suggested arsenic requirement for animals is between 25 and 50 ng As/g (based on diets containing 4000 kcal/kg). Extrapolated to the human population, this dietary intake is equal to 12.5 to 25 µg As/day. Human diets normally contain 12 to 50 µg As/day, and thus the postulated arsenic requirement for humans apparently can be met by food and water normally consumed. However, there may be dietary situations where the requirement for arsenic is not met (for example, low dietary arsenic coupled with an altered methionine metabolism or hemodialysis).

Food sources. Arsenic (inorganic and organic) in the diet is contributed by various foods including cereals and breads, 18.1 per cent; starchy vegetables, 14.9 per cent; and meats and fish, 32.1 per cent. About 20 per cent of the daily intake of arsenic is inorganic. Arsenic in water is almost all inorganic and most drinking water contains less than 10 µg As/L and, typically, 2 to 3 µg/L. Drinking water can contribute 20 µg inorganic As/day.

Toxicity. Toxicity of organic arsenicals, including compounds such as monomethylarsonic acid, dimethylarsenic acid, arsenobetaine, and arsenocholine, is low. Inorganic forms are more toxic than organic forms of arsenic; generally arsenite (+3) is more toxic than arsenate (+5). Signs of inorganic arsenic toxicity include dermatosis, hematopoietic depression, liver damage, sensory disturbances, peripheral neuritis, anorexia, and skin and internal cancers.

Biotin

Biotin is also known as vitamin H and coenzyme R (Hexahydro-2-oxo-1H-thienal [3, 4-d]- imidazole-4-pentatonic acid). It is found primarily in liver, kidney and muscle. Biotin functions as an essential cofactor for four carboxylases that catalyze the incorporation of cellular bicarbonate into the carbon backbone of organic compounds. Acetyl-CoA carboxylase (ACC) is located in the cytosol where it catalyzes the formation of malonyl-CoA which then serves as a substrate for fatty acid elongation. The other three enzymes are located in the mitochondria. Pyruvate carboxylase (PC) catalyzes the incorporation of bicarbonate into pyruvate to form oxaloacetate, an intermediate in the tricarboxylic acid cycle. In gluconeogenic tissues such as the liver and kidney, oxaloacetate can be converted to glucose. Methcrotonyl-CoA carboxylase (MCC) catalyzes the incorporation of bicarbonate into propionyl-CoA to form methylmalonyl-CoA which, in turn, is metabolized to other compounds that eventually enter the tricarboxylic acid cycle.

Deficiencies. Severe deficiency causes (1) thinning of hair, loss of hair color, and eventually complete loss of hair; (2) a scaly, red rash distributed around the openings of the eyes, nose, mouth, and perineal area; and (3) central nervous system abnormalities such as depression, lethargy, hallucinations, and paresthesias. In infants, the neurologic findings include hypotonia, lethargy, and developmental delay, as well as a peculiar withdrawn behaviour. In patients on total or near total intravenous feeding, an unusual distribution of facial fat coupled with the rash and hair loss produces a distinct appearance called "biotin deficiency facies."

Clinical uses. Biotin is routinely provided to individuals receiving total intravenous feeding and is incorporated into almost all nutritionally complete dietary supplements and infant formulas. In larger doses, biotin is also used to treat inborn errors of metabolism such as biotinidase deficiency, holocarboxylase synthetase deficiency, and the isolated deficiencies of PC, PCC, and MCC. Marginal states of biotin deficiency may develop during normal pregnancy, possibly due to accelerated biotin breakdown. Adequate intakes for pregnancy may need to be revised upward in the future; however, no untoward effects of marginal biotin status in pregnancy have been proven to date. Marginal status has also been detected in patients taking anticonvulsants; these anticonvulsants appear to accelerate the rate of biotin breakdown and interfere with biotin absorption.

Diet recommendations. The estimated safe and adequate dietary intake values for biotin for different age groups are as follows: 5, 6, 8, 12, 20, 25 and 30 ug/day for ages of 0-0.5, 0.5-1, 1-3, 4-8, 9-13, 14-18 and >19 years, respectively. The values for pregnacy and lactation were estimated to be 30 and 35 ug/day, respectively.

Food sources. Biotin is widely distributed in food stuffs, but the amounts are small relative to other vitamins. Biotin deficiency is rare in the absence of total intravenous feedings without added biotin or the chronic ingestion of raw egg white.

Toxicity. Oral and intravenous doses up to 200 mg have not produced frank toxicity in human subjects. In animal studies, even higher doses per kilogram body weight have not produced toxicity.

Boron

Boron (B) is a trace mineral that is essential for plants. Boron may also be essential for humans and animals based on recent experimental evidence showing that boron affects blood biochemical markers of energy and mineral metabolism. Specifically, boron seems to be important for energy utilization and the development and maintenance of bone.

Deficiencies. In vitamin D deficient animals fed very low intakes of boron there were increases in total calcium loss, interference with the use of blood sugar (glucose), fat, and insulin, and dminished bone development. In humans, no deficiencies have been documented in free-living populations. However, careful study of volunteers in special living quarters shows that reducing the amount of dietary boron causes changes in blood glucose and fat similar to that seen in boron-deficient animals.

For reasons not fully understood, boron supplementation increases the percent of calcium intake lost in the urine of both pre- and post-menopausal volunteers. Very low intakes of boron may aggravate the symptoms of arthritis.

Diet recommendations. The usual adult dietary boron intake in the US is about 1 mg/day. Use of boron supplements is not recommended because neither an Estimated Safe and Adequate Dietary Intake (ESADDI) or Recommended Daily Allowance (RDA) has been set for boron.

Food sources. The main sources of boron in the diet are drinking water (which varies considerably between geographical locations), milk and dairy products, and juices and beverages. On a wet weight basis, fruits, vegetables, legumes and nuts (dicotyledonous plants) contain much more boron than grains, breads, and cereals (monocotyledonous plants). Animal products (meats, poultry, fish, etc.) contain very little boron but milk and dairy products are major contributors to total boron intake because of the large quantities consumed.

Toxicity. Almost all the boron that enters the body from diet or absorption through damaged skin is promptly excreted in the urine. However, this control process can be overwhelmed by very high boron intakes that cause acute boron toxicity with nausea, vomiting, headache, diarrhea, hypothermia, restlessness, skin loss, kidney damage, and death from circulatory collapse and shock. The minimum lethal dose for humans is not known although single doses of 18 to 20 g in adults have been fatal. Chronic boron toxicity symptoms include poor appetite, nausea, weight loss, and decreased sexual activity, seminal volume, and sperm count. Death from boron poisoning is rare probably because of the emphasis placed on maintaining electrolytic balance and supporting kidney function during the worst part of the illness.

Calcium

Calcium is the most common mineral in the human body. Calcium is a nutrient in the news because adequate intakes are an important determinant of bone health and risk of fracture or osteoporosis. Our nation suffers from approximately 1.5 million fractures annually with an associated health care cost of $13.8 billion.

Approximately 99% of total body calcium is in the skeleton and teeth and 1% in blood and soft tissues. Calcium has four major biological functions: (1) structural as stores in the skeleton, (2) electrophysiological - carries charge during an action potential across membranes, (3) intracellular regulator, and (4) as a cofactor for extracellular enzymes and regulatory proteins. Calcium is present in variable amounts in all the foods and water we consume, although the main sources are dairy products and vegetables.

Deficiencies. Acute deficiency symptoms are avoided because of the large skeletal stores. Prolonged bone resorption from chronic dietary deficiency results in osteoporosis either by inadequate accumulation of bone mass during growth or increased rate of bone loss at menopause. Dietary calcium deficiency also has been associated with increased risk of hypertension, preeclampsia, and colon cancer.

Dietary recommendations. The dietary recommendations set by the 1997 National Academy of Science Panel on Calcium and Related Nutrients are: 210 mg/d for 0-6 month olds, 270 mg/d for 6-12 month olds, 500 mg/d for 1-3 year olds, 800 mg/d for 4-8 year olds, 1300 mg/d for individuals aged 9-18 years, 1000 mg/d for individuals aged 19-50 years, and 1200 mg/d for individuals over the age of 51 years. No alterations for pregnancy or lactation were recommended. The recommended upper level of calcium is 2.5 g/day.

Food sources. Dairy products are the most concentrated, well-absorbed sources of calcium. Few other foods are rich sources of calcium. Foods which can contribute to dietary calcium include firm tofu (chemically set with calcium), dried beans, kale, broccoli, and bok choy. Calcium from oxalate rich foods such as spinach is generally poorly absorbed. Phytates are slightly inhibitory to absorption. Since FDA allows a label claim relating calcium to prevention of osteoporosis, some fortified foods have become available on the market.

Toxicity. Symptoms of calcium toxicity are largely anecdotal. Excess calcium supplementation has been associated with some mineral imbalances such as zinc.

Carbohydrates

Carbohydrates are the principal dietary source of energy. They are comprised of simple sugars and complex carbohydrates. The most common simple sugars, or monosaccharides (i.e., one sugar unit) include glucose, fructose, galactose and mannose. Glucose is the main form in which carbohydrate is absorbed, exchanged between tissues, and channeled into metabolic pathways. One molecule of glucose contains 6 atoms of carbon, 6 atoms of oxygen and 12 atoms of hydrogen. The name carbohydrates (often abbreviated as 'CHO') derives from the fact that these compounds are primarily made up of carbon atoms and water. Disaccharides (i.e., two sugar units) include sucrose (also called saccharose), maltose and lactose. Oligosaccharides, such as raffinose and stachyose in legumes, are composed of 3-10 sugars. Polysaccharides are substances in which multiple, often hundreds of monosaccharides molecules, are linked together. The most abundant edible forms are the starches present in grains, potatoes, etc., which are polymers of glucose. The two major forms of these complex carbohydrates are amylose and amylopectin. In animals, the storage form of carbohydrates is glycogen. Dextrins are fragments of starch produced by dry heat, such as toasting.

Dietary fibers such as cellulose are polysaccharides in which glucose or other monosaccharides are linked by bonds which cannot be hydrolysed by the digestive enzymes produced in the intestine. Dietary fiber, dextrins and some oligosaccharides are thus not digestible, except through the action of enzymes produced by intestinal bacteria. Undigested dietary fiber passes to the large bowel where it is fermented by bacteria to yield lactic acid and the short-chain fatty acids acetic, propionic and butyric acid. Humans derive measurable amounts of energy from the metabolism of these products of bacterial fermentation. This process is very active in herbivores which can thereby derive most of their energy from cellulose. Other carbohydrate-related compounds include polyols (i.e., sugar alcohols such as sorbitol and xylitol) and organic acids, such as ascorbic acid (i.e., vitamin C), citric acid and malic acid. Although monosaccharide yield slightly less energy than starches (3.7 vs. 4.2 kilocalories per g), the energy value of dietary carbohydrates is generally considered to be an even 4 kilocalories per gram.

Deficiency. There is no absolute requirement for dietary carbohydrate, although the brain, the red blood cells and some cells in the kidney use glucose as a preferred source of energy. The liver has a considerable capacity to synthesize glucose from amino acids (from dietary and body protein) and glycerol, released from lipid hydrolysis. When intake of dietary sugars and starch is low or lacking, stored fat (triacyglyceride) is mobilized, providing fatty acids to sustain energy generation in the body. A carbohydrate-free diet is associated with increased protein breakdown and ketone body formation in the liver, which may produce dehydration and loss of cations, though not to the same dangerous extent as in diabetic ketoacidosis. Starvation ketosis is greatly attenuated by daily intakes of as little as 50-100 g of carbohydrate.

Diet recommendations. No formal diet recommendation for carbohydrates exists as intakes are adequate in US diets, though consumption of some 25 grams of dietary fiber (i.e. undigestible polysaccharides) is recommended. The Daily Value for carbohydrates used in nutritional labeling is 60% of total calories, or 300 g/day for a 2,000 Calorie diet. In 1985, the US average carbohydrate intake was 177 g in women and 287 g in men. Approximately 23% came from fruits and vegetables and 41% was from grain products. About half of the carbohydrate intake was in the form of mono- and disaccharides and the reminder as complex carbohydrates.

Food sources. Monosaccharides such as glucose and fructose are found in fruits and honey. Sucrose (glucose linked to fructose), or table sugar (produced from sugar cane or sugar beets) is the most commonly consumed disaccharide, found also in molasses, maple syrup and some fruits. Maltose (two glucose units) is a component of sprouting grains, malted cereals and syrups. By converting the glucose in corn syrups into fructose, isosyrups with increased sweetening power are produced which are used instead of cane sugar, notably in confectionary items and soft drinks. Lactose (a dissacharide of glucose and galactose) is the sugar in milk. Amylose is the dominant starch in wheat and rice. Amylopectin is found in corn, potatoes and tapioca.

Resistant starches are starches which are poorly digested in the human gastrointestinal tract, either because the starch is in granular form (e.g., uncooked) and therefore resistant to digestive enzymes, or in the form of retrograded amylose, which may form after cooling starch that has been gelatinized by moist heating. Up to 7-10% of starch from wheat, oats and potatoes and 20% from baked beans can pass through to the colon. Resistant starches which reach the colon are fermented there by the microflora and converted into short-chain fatty acids, a process which also yields small amounts of methane gas and hydrogen.

Recent research. Conversion of carbohydrate into fat allows animals to build up fat reserves even when their feed contains very little fat. It has therefore long been believed that excess carbohydrate can readily be converted into stored body fat. However, it is now well established that in man, fat synthesis is essentially negligible under conditions of unrestricted access to food. On another front, it has been shown recently that hyperactivity in children is not associated with sugar intake. Of continued major interest are studies on the beneficial effect of consuming more complex carbohydrates which have a relatively low glycemic index (i.e., they cause a less abrupt increase in blood glucose levels after meals) instead of the more rapidly absorbed sugars and starches. This is particularly important for individuals affected by insulin-dependent, as well as non-insulin dependent, diabetes mellitus and because complex carbohydrates tend to exert favorable effects on blood lipid levels in subjects at risk for cardiovascular disease. In addition there is continuing research into the role of non-starch polysaccharides (fiber) in the prevention of colonic cancer.

Toxicity. Ingestion of even large amounts of carbohydrates has no adverse effects, except that lactose-containing milk products can lead to diarrhea in lactase-deficient populations. In individuals affected by certain inherited carbohydrate-metabolizing enzyme deficiencies, carbohydrate intake may have to be carefully controlled to avoid possibly severe adverse reactions.

Carnitine

L-Carnitine (L-?-hydroxy-? -N, N, N-trimethylaminobutyric acid) is a non-essential organic nutrient required for entry of long-chain fatty acids (as acylcarnitine esters) into mitochondria. It also facilitates removal of short-chain organic acids from mitochondria, thereby freeing intramitochondrial coenzyme A to participate in the ?-oxidation and tricarboxylic acid cycle pathways. Carnitine is a substrate for carnitine palmitoyltransferases I and II and carnitine acetyltransferase, enzymes that participate in and regulate fatty acid utilization. Carnitine and its esters are transported across the inner mitochondrial membrane specifically by carnitine-acylcarnitine translocase. The D-isomer of carnitine is biologically inactive. Carnitine is concentrated in most tissues of the body, with about 97% in skeletal muscle. L-Carnitine is synthesized from the essential amino acids lysine and methionine. In humans, the last enzymatic reaction in the pathway occurs primarily in liver and kidney, but not in skeletal and heart muscle. The normal rate of carnitine synthesis in humans is 0.16 to 0.48 mg/kg body weight/day.

Deficiencies. Carnitine deficiency occurs as a primary genetic defect of carnitine transport and secondary to a variety of genetic and acquired disorders. These disorders often are associated with fasting hypoglycemia, lethargy and cardiomyopathy. A murine model of systemic carnitine deficiency (the jvs mouse) has been studied in some detail. Reports of nutritional carnitine deficiency are rare, and in the few cases described, other genetic causes were not specifically excluded. Infants are particularly susceptible to carnitine depletion, because the demands of tissue accretion associated with rapid growth exceed the ability of the infant to synthesize carnitine. However, the substantially lower plasma carnitine concentrations (and, presumably, lower tissue carnitine concentrations) do not impair growth rates or other indicators of normal development.

Diet recommendations. Carnitine is not required in the diet of normal humans. Daily intakes of omnivores and strict vegetarians are 20 mg to 200 mg and <1 mg for a 70 kg (154 lb.) person, respectively. Infant formulas (including total parenteral nutrition solutions) that do not contain carnitine (e.g., non-milk-based formulas) should be supplemented with carnitine to the levels found in human milk, 11.3 mg/L (70 mmol/L).

Food sources. Red meats are the best sources of carnitine (50 to 120 mg/100 g). Fish, chicken and milk are good sources (1.6 to 6.4 mg/100 g). Vegetables, fruits, grains, and other plant-derived foods contain very little carnitine (<0.05 mg/100 g). Approximately 65 to 75 per cent of dietary carnitine is absorbed. Unabsorbed carnitine is almost entirely degraded by bacteria in the large intestine. No dietary components are known to impair absorption. There is no known toxicity associated with ingestion from normal dietary components. Supplements that provide more than 3,000 mg (19 mmol) of carnitine per day may cause diarrhea and/or "fish odor" syndrome.

Carotenoids

There are over 600 carotenoids in nature. Carotenoids generally contain a conjugated polyene structure which is efficient at absorbing light, and are the major yellow and red pigments in many fruits and vegetables. Beta-carotene (C40 H56) and alpha-carotene are responsible for the orange color of carrots, and lycopene for the red color of tomatoes; astaxanthin imparts a red or pink color to lobsters and salmon. The term "carotene" refers to carotenoids which contain only carbon and hydrogen (e.g. beta-carotene, alpha-carotene, lycopene), while the term "xanthophylls" refers to compounds which contain hydroxyl groups (lutein, zeaxanthin, beta-cryptoxanthin) or keto groups (canthaxanthin) or both (astaxanthin).

Major storage sites. Because the carotenoids are fat-soluble, they are found in fatty tissues in the body and are transported in blood by lipoproteins. The predominant carotenoids found in human tissues are beta-carotene, alpha-carotene, lycopene, lutein, zeaxanthin, and beta-cryptoxanthin; their relative abundance depends on dietary intake.

Functions. In animals some carotenoids (particularly beta-carotene) serve as dietary precursors to vitamin A, and many of them may function as fat-soluble antioxidants. Because they are present in much lower concentrations than is alpha-tocopherol, some questions have been raised about their physiological importance as antioxidants. However, increased consumption of foods rich in carotenoids is associated with decreased risk of some degenerative diseases, and there is some evidence also for their role in improving immune function. In plants they serve as antioxidants to protect the highly reactive photosystems and also act as accessory photopigments.

Deficiency. One study has found that carotenoid deficiency is associated with skin changes (including acne and dermatitis). These changes were detrimental but not life-threatening. This effect should be confirmed by additional studies before making dietary recommendations.

Diet recommendations. No formal diet recommendation for carotenoids has yet been established but some experts suggest intakes of 5 to 6 mg daily (about twice the average daily American intake). Individual dietary carotenoid consumption is quite variable.

Food sources. Carotenoids are biosynthesized only in plants and some bacteria, thus foods of plant origin are the primary dietary source for humans. Intestinal absorption can be poor, and depends on the presence of dietary fat. Mild cooking (steaming) increases bioavailability of carotenoids while overcooking can destroy some forms. The extent of conversion of provitamin A carotenoids to vitamin A seems to be variable but is less than 50 per cent.

Toxicity. The carotenoids are remarkably devoid of toxicity, and serve as good nontoxic sources of vitamin A. Massive overconsumption of carotenoids can result in yellowing of the skin, especially of the hand and ears (xanthosis cutis), but has no adverse health effects. The color disappears within a week or so after reducing intake of carotene-rich foods.

Clinical uses. Canthaxanthin and beta-carotene have been used pharmacologically to treat erythropoietic porphyria, a disease characterized by extreme sensitivity of the skin to sunlight.

Chloride

Chloride is an anion generally consumed as sodium chloride (NaCl) or table salt. There is a high correlation between the sodium and chloride contents of the diet, and only under unusual circumstances do levels of sodium and chloride vary in the diet independently. Adequate intake of sodium chloride is required for maintenance of extracellular fluid volume. Chloride is both actively and passively absorbed. Urine excretion reflects chloride intake, with low or no chloride found in deficiency states.

In general chloride has received little attention in dietary assessment and has been omitted from food composition tables. However, chloride content of infant cow's milk and soy formulae has stimulated interest in the past 15 years because of iatrogenic hypochloremia induced by several infant formulas with deficient chloride concentrations.

Deficiencies. An adequate intake of sodium chloride to sustain losses may result in hypotension. Depending on intake of "free" water, hyponatremia and hypochloremia may ensue, such as in water overload, wasting, and trauma with sequestration of extracellular fluid as in burns. Selective chloride deficiency (without sodium deficiency) may result from vomiting, as in pyloric stenosis in infancy or continuous gastric suction with resulting metabolic alkalosis. A familial autosomal recessive condition with chronic diarrhea and defective chloride reabsorption (Barter's Syndrome) also causes hypochloremia. Renal tubular disorders, cystic fibrosis with excessive sweating and loss of chloride in the perspiration and diuretic use may also cause low chloride states. As mentioned above, inadvertent feeding of chloride deficient infant formulae (<5 mEq Cl/L) resulted in 141 infants in the first year of life developing failure-to-thrive, anorexia, weakness and some ambiguous findings of slow development. Deficiency of chloride alone leads to contraction of extracellular fluid volume and metabolic alkalosis which, in turn, leads to a deficiency of potassium by increasing urinary excretion of potassium.

Diet recommendations. High sodium, low chloride diets should be avoided. In the absence of sodium chloride losing disorders (e.g., excessive sweating, cystic fibrosis, Addison's disease) several health agencies have recommended that the general population not consume more than 6 g NaCl/day. This recommendation may be of benefit in decreasing cardiovascular morbidity and mortality associated with higher levels of blood pressure in the resting stat. The minimal daily requirement for sodium chloride for normal individuals is less than 2 g NaCl/ day. For chloride alone, the Estimated Minimum Requirements per day set by the Food and Nutrition Board are as follows: infants: 0-6 months, 180 mg; 6 months-11 months, 300 mg; 1 year, 350 mg; 2-5 years, 500 mg; 6-9 years, 600 mg; and adolescents and adults, 750 mg.

Food sources. With few exceptions (e.g., monosodium glutamate and sodium bicarbonate) sodium and chloride are most often consumed as sodium chloride (salt). Human milk contains about 420 mg/L and infant formula is now required to contain 55-65 mg/100 kcal and is not to exceed 150 mg/100 kcal. Undiluted cow's milk contains about 900-1020 mg/L. Infant formula contains 10.6-13.5 m Eq/L and formula for older infants (follow-up formula), 14-19.2 m Eq/L. Recommended intakes are 2-4 m Eq/L/Kg for infants and children and 60-150 m Eq (total) adolescents.

Choline

Choline, a dietary component of many foods, is part of several major phospholipids (including phosphatidylcholine - also called lecithin) that are critical for normal membrane structure and function. The major precursor of betaine, it is used by the kidney to maintain water balance and by the liver as a source of methyl-groups for methionine formation. Also, choline is used to produce the important neurotransmitter acetylcholine. In the body choline is mainly found in phospholipids, such as lecithin (phosphatidylcholine) and sphingomyelin. The outer leaflet of plasma membrane is rich in these choline-phospholipids whereas the inner leaflet is dominated by phosphatidylethanolamine, phosphatidylserine and phosphatidylinositol. Phosphatidylcholine, the predominant phospholipid (>50%) in most mammalian membranes, not only contributes to the structure of the membrane bilayer, but products of receptor-mediated lecithin hydrolysis also serve as important second messengers in signal cascades that control cell growth and gene expression. Disaturated phosphatidylcholine is the primary active component of surfactant in the lung; a deficiency of surfactant in the neonate leads to respiratory distress syndrome in premature infants.

The metabolism of choline, methionine, and methyl-folate are closely interrelated; the metabolic pathways intersect at the formation of methionine from homocysteine. Some choline can be formed from methionine (through the methylation of phosphatidylethanolamine by phosphatidylethanolamine N-methyltransferase using S-adenosylmethionine as the methyl donor). This can provide some of the choline required by humans.

There are a number of mechanisms that ensure the developing fetus and the infant receive adequate amounts of choline. Like other nutrients, large amounts of choline are delivered to the fetus across the placenta. This depletes maternal stores of choline. Human milk is an especially good source of choline.

Deficiencies. Although each of the above functions is absolutely vital for the maintenance of normal cellular and organ functions, it has been difficult to identify choline-deficiency syndromes in humans. The Institute of Medicine noted that "Healthy males with normal folate and vitamin B_{12} status fed a choline deficient diet have diminished plasma choline and phosphatidylcholine concentrations, and develop liver damage. For these humans, de novo synthesis of choline was not adequate to meet the demand for the nutrient." Patients fed by total parenteral nutrition sometimes develop fatty liver, abnormal liver function tests, and low plasma choline and phosphatidylcholine concentrations. This is in part due to an impaired capacity to de novo synthesize choline. In some of these patients, these abnormalities resolve when they are treated with a dietary source of choline.

Diet recommendations. Based on the limited human data that is currently available, the Institute of Medicine, National Academy of Sciences USA, recommended that humans consume choline. They set an adequate intake (AI) level for choline of 550 mg/day for men and 425 mg/day for women. For children, the AI was proportionately adjusted for body size.

Food sources. Choline and choline esters can be found in significant amounts in many foods consumed by humans; some of the choline is added during processing (especially in the preparation of infant formula). Little reference information exists on the relative choline content of foods, but we estimate the average choline dietary intake (as choline and choline esters) of the adult human to be more than 500 mg/day. Orally ingested choline (e.g., as hydrochloride salt) may be degraded by intestinal bacteria and cause a fishy body odor; this does not occur when lecithin is eaten.

Clinical uses. Amino acid-glucose solutions used in total parenteral nutrition of humans lack choline. The lipid emulsions that deliver extra calories and essential fatty acids during parenteral nutrition contain choline in the form of lecithin (20 per cent emulsion contains 13.2 mmol/L). Humans treated with parenteral nutrition required 1-1.7 mmol of choline-containing phospholipid/day during the first week of parenteral nutrition therapy to maintain plasma choline levels.

There are no established approaches to determine nutritional status for choline. Plasma choline and phosphatidylcholine concentrations fall when humans are fed a choline-deficient diet or after strenuous, prolonged physical activity, such as running a marathon. Even in severe deficiency, plasma choline concentrations do not fall below 50 per cent of normal. Measurement of serum alanine aminotransferase activity, which rises approximately 1 week after the feeding a choline-deficient diet, may prove beneficial in assessment of choline nutritional status.

Toxicity. Large oral doses of choline or phosphatidylcholine may be associated with hypotension, sweating, salivation and diarrhea. Large doses of choline can cause a fishy body odor.

The Tolerable Upper Limit for adults has been set at 3.5 g/day of choline.

Chromium

Chromium (Cr) is an essential nutrient required for normal sugar and fat metabolism. Chromium functions primarily by potentiating the action of insulin. Chromium occurs primarily in the trivalent and hexavalent forms; the form in higher organisms is trivalent. This mineral occurs throughout the body with highest concentrations in the liver, kidney, spleen and bone.

Deficiency. Signs of deficiency include impaired glucose tolerance and elevated circulating insulin. In some studies, chromium supplementation has reduced total serum cholesterol, triglycerides and apolipoprotein B and increased HDL-cholesterol.

Diet recommendations. The Estimated Safe and Adequate Daily Dietary Intake (ESADDI) for adults is 50 to 200 μg. Usual dietary intakes in the U.S. are about 25 μg/day for women and 33 μg/day for men. Breast-fed infants consume less than 1 μg Cr/day and the ESADDI for infants is 10 to 40 μg/day. The current ESADDI for chromium needs to be re-evaluated.

Food sources/bioavailability. Meat, poultry, fish and dairy products are generally low in chromium. Fruits, vegetables whole grains and seeds are better sources but have variable concentrations. Processing foods with stainless steel equipment may increase their chromium concentration, especially if the foods are acidic. In addition, there are differences in bioavailability and biological activity of the different complexes found in foods.

Toxicity. Both solubility and oxidation state affect the potential for toxicity; furthermore, the type of complex may impact toxicity. Toxic effects are limited primarily to industrial exposure to hexavalent chromium, which is much more toxic than the trivalent form. The hexavalent chromium compounds may be carcinogenic. The acidity of the stomach promotes reduction of hexavalent chromium to the trivalent form. Most of the chromium absorbed from the gastrointestinal tract is trivalent. The Reference Dose (RfD) for trivalent chromium is 1 mg/kg/day. This level is more than 300-fold the upper limit of the ESADDI, making trivalent chromium one of the least toxic nutrients.

Copper

Copper (Cu) is a trace element that is essential for most animals, including humans. The influence of copper upon human health is due to the fact it is part of enzymes, which are proteins that help biochemical reactions occur in every cell. Copper is involved in the absorption, storage and metabolism of iron. The symptoms of a copper deficiency are similar to iron deficiency anemia. Copper may be absorbed by both the stomach and small intestinal mucosa, with most absorbed by the small intestine. Copper is found in the blood bound to proteins.

Copper is utilized by most cells as a component of enzymes involved in energy production (cytochrome oxidase) and in the protection of cells from free radical damage (superoxide dismutase). Copper is also involved with an enzyme that strengthens connective tissue (lysyl oxidase) and in brain neurotransmitters (dopamine hydroxylase and peptidyl alpha amidating monoxygenase). One of the proteins, ceruloplasmin, transports copper as well as helps convert iron to a form that can be transported to other tissues. The average level of copper stored in the body is from 50 to 120 mg, with most of this in the liver. Excess dietary copper can also lead to high copper levels in the kidney. However, under normal situations, not much copper is excreted via the urine. Most copper is excreted via bile that is released into the gastrointestinal tract, with minimal copper reabsorbed by intestinal cells. The uptake of copper and elimination through the bile allows copper to be conserved and tightly regulated.

Deficiencies. Animals that are fed diets deficient in copper often exhibit anemia, cardiac abnormalities such as blood vessel and heart rupture, abnormal EKG's and have elevated levels of serum cholesterol, triglycerides and glucose. A lifetime of marginal diet copper in humans is thought to lead to heart disease. Copper deficiency has been observed in premature infants and infants suffering from malnutrition. Overt symptoms in adults are rare, but may occur with long term shortage or, possibly, in those who consume zinc supplements for a period of time.

Diet recommendations. The estimated safe and adequate intake for copper is 1.5 - 3.0 mg/day. Many survey studies show that Americans consume about 1.0 mg or less of copper per day. Copper is found in foods such as nuts [0.2 to 0.5 mg/28 g (1 Tbsp.)], shellfish (1.0 to 3.7 mg/serving), organ meats (3.8 mg/serving of beef liver) and legumes (0.2 mg/serving). Grains, grain products and chocolate have appreciable levels of copper. While these food items are good to excellent sources of copper, the absolute amount of copper absorbed may be influenced by other dietary components.

Copper absorption may be decreased by excess dietary iron or zinc. Conversely, too much copper may cause an iron deficiency. Vitamin C supplementation results in decreased copper status. In rats, large doses of vitamin C can lead to copper deficiency. Other dietary components have an influence upon copper status, but not necessarily absorption. Feeding rats either sucrose or fructose, as opposed to glucose or cornstarch, decreases copper status and exacerbates the signs of copper deficiency.

Toxicity. Cases of copper toxicity are rare but may occur. Excess copper consumption may lead to liver damage. Intake of supplements exceeding 3 mg copper/day for a protracted period of time may be cause for concern. Doses of 10 mg/day over several weeks may lead to toxic symptoms, such as weakness and nausea.

Genetic Conditions relating to copper. There are two well known genetic diseases affecting copper metabolism. Menkes' kinky-hair disease is a problem with copper transport or absorption. Wilson's disease is characterized by increased liver copper content, leading to severe hepatic damage, followed by increased brain copper levels and neurological problems. Menkes' disease results in pathology resembling copper-deficiency, as opposed to the pathology of Wilson's disease, which resembles copper-toxicity. The Menkes' gene codes for a P-type ATPase that has a mutation that prevents copper absorption in the intestine.

Energy

Energy is required for the functions of all biological systems. Dietary energy is commonly given in units of Calories or kilocalories, but the acceptable scientific terminology is joules. The primary sources of dietary energy are fats, carbohydrates and protein. Ethanol also contributes dietary energy in individuals consuming alcoholic beverages, but alcohol is not generally categorized as a nutrient. The energy for biological processes is obtained from these sources by intermediary metabolism. Our bodies are very efficient in storing energy for future use. Stored energy is primarily in the form of fat in adipose tissue, but a small amount of carbohydrate is stored in the liver and muscle as glycogen. Intermediary metabolism converts the energy consumed into the forms for storage or into forms which are readily available for biological processes such as compounds with high energy phosphate bonds.

Since energy cannot be destroyed or created, over a period of time the energy consumed must be expended or accounted for by gains or losses in body tissues. If energy intakes are less then expenditures, body weight loss will occur. When energy intakes exceed expenditures, body weight gain will occur. There is evidence of adaptive responses to fluctuations in energy intake which are dependent of genetic and environmental factors. While these adaptations may account for some of the variability between individuals, they do not prevent body weight changes in response to unbalanced energy equations. Energy expenditures are based on: Energy Needs = Basal metabolic rate (energy to keep heart beating, etc.) + physical activity + Thermic effect of feeding (energy for intermediary metabolism).

Diet recommendations. Recommended dietary allowances for energy are based on Median Heights and Weights set by the Food and Nutrition Board. The average energy allowance for infants (0.5-1.0 years, 9 kg or 20 lb, 71 cm or 28 in) is 98 kcal/kg or 850 kcal/day. The average energy allowance for children (4-6 years, 20 kg or 44 lb, 112 cm or 44 in) is 90 kcal/kg or 1,800 kcal/day. The average energy allowance for males (11-14 years, 45 kg or 99 lb, 157 cm or 62 in) is 55 kcal/Kg or 2,500 kcal/day. The average energy allowance for males (25-50 years,

79 kg or 174 lb, 176 cm or 70 in) is 37 kcal/kg or 2,900 kcal/day. The average energy allowance for females (11-14 years, 46 kg or 101 lb, 157 cm or 62 in) is 47 kcal/kg or 2,200 kcal/day. The average energy allowance for females (25-50 years, 63 kg or 138 lb, 163 cm or 64 in) is 36 kcal/kg or 2,200 kcal/day. There is wide variation in individuals' energy requirements, primarily because of differences in body size and physical activity. The energy allowances above are for individuals with median heights and weights, and light to moderate activity levels. The recommended allowances should be adjusted to account for increased physical activity and for larger or smaller body size.

Inadequate energy intakes. Starvation continues to be a major world problem. Fortunately, starvation because of inadequate food availability is almost unheard of in the US. However, self imposed starvation is recognized in a proportion of people in the US with anorexia nervosa.

Excessive energy intakes. Obesity is a major health problem in developed countries in the world. It has been estimated that 25-35% of the US adult population is obese. Obesity is associated with increased risk for cardiovascular disease, hypertension, stroke, diabetes and for certain cancers (endometrial, colon, ovarian and breast).

Fiber

Dietary fiber includes a variety of plant-derived compounds, i.e., non-starch polysaccharides and lignin, that are not digested by endogenous intestinal enzymes. Fiber is composed of a variety of materials that are often categorized as insoluble or soluble in boiling water. Insoluble polysaccharides include cellulose and some forms of hemicellulose. Lignin is part of insoluble fiber that is not a polysaccharide but a polymer of phenylpropane molecules. The soluble fibers include pectins, gums, and mucilages.

Fiber is neither digested nor absorbed in the small intestine but is fermented by bacteria in the colon. On a typical American diet, about 75 per cent of ingested fiber is fermented. While there is no absolute requirement for dietary fiber, it is almost certainly needed for normal bowel function. Adequate fiber clearly prevents constipation, diverticular disease of the colon, and hemorrhoids. Many other physiologic effects have been attributed to fiber and consumption of diets high in fiber may prevent a variety of conditions including obesity, diabetes, gallstones, coronary artery disease, or colon cancer. Epidemiological studies show fairly clearly that diets high in fruits, vegetables and cereal grains are associated with decreased risk of developing these diseases.

Diet recommendations. Current average fiber intake is estimated at about 12 g/day. Many health organizations recommend 20-35 g/day but there is no level set in the current Recommended Dietary Allowances.

Food sources. Foods that are rich in dietary fiber include whole grains (particularly the bran portions), legumes, and some fruits and vegetables. Most foods contain mixtures of both insoluble and soluble fiber. Examples of foods rich in insoluble fiber are wheat bran, nuts and barley; soluble fiber is found in oat bran, melons, and dried fruits. Beans are good sources of both fiber types. Cooking does not decrease the amount of fiber in food but changes its three-dimensional structure.

Potential hazards. There are some concerns that phytate, which accompanies dietary fiber, will decrease the absorption of certain minerals like iron, calcium, magnesium, and manganese. However, most long term studies have not confirmed this danger. Very high intakes of isolated sources of dietary fiber can prevent adequate intake of other nutrients and may, in rare instances, lead to intestinal obstruction or volvulus of the colon. Most untoward effects have been traced to inadequate fluid intake with consumption of large amounts of fiber, usually in a purified form. This indicates the desirability of obtaining fiber from food sources, rather than from supplements.

Flouride

The trace element fluorine is present in the body almost entirely in bone and teeth. Because of its high reactivity, fluorine exists as its anion fluoride. Fluoride's best known effect is to serve as a catalyst for both the mineralization of developing tooth enamel prior to tooth eruption and for remineralization of surface enamel. The combination of these fluoride effects greatly reduces occurrence of dental decay (caries). Denotal caries is an infectious disease caused by bacteria. When food is ingested, oral bacteria multiply within their home (plaque) and produce organic acids. Loss of tooth enamel accelerates as long as plaque pH is less than 5.5. The presence of fluoride changes some of the tooth crystal into a less acid-soluble crystal known as fluoropatite.

Diet recommendations. The Food and Nutrition Board of the National Academy of Sciences has concluded that a fluoride intake of 0.05 mg/kg body weight, after the age of 6 months, provides an adequate fluoride intake to reduce risk of dental decay. It is assumed that this fluoride will come from a combination of food and water sources.

Food sources. The major source of fluoride is drinking water. Seafood, some teas, and foods made with mechanically separated chicken (baby food, canned meats, luncheon meats, and frankfurters) contribute to total fluoride intake. Otherwise, most foods are very low in fluoride.

Clinical uses. Regular comsumption of fluoride from a community water supply plus regular use of fluoridated toothpaste can significantly decrease prevalence of dental decay. Dietary fluoride supplements are only recommended for children when the water supplies fluoride at less than 0.3 mg/L. In this case, fluoride supplements of 0.25 mg/day for ages 0.5-3 years, 0.5 mg/day for ages 3-6 years, and 1 mg/day for ages 6-16 years can be recommended. No dietary fluoride supplement is recommended when water supplies fluoride at greater than 0.6 mg/L.

Under controlled experimental conditions, slow release administration of fluoride (23 mg/day) plus calcium has been shown to stimulate new bone formation in some individuals.

Toxicity. Children less than 8 years of age can develop mottled tooth enamel (white horizontal lines with hypo-mineralized areas susceptable to decay in extreme cases) if they ingest several times more fluoride than recommended during tooth enamel formation. Swallowing of fluoridated toothpaste by young children has been shown to be the most prevalent cause of this problem.

Iron

Iron (Fe) is an essential nutrient that carries oxygen and forms part of the oxygen-carrying proteins, hemoglobin in red blood cells and myoglobin in muscle. It is also a necessary component of various enzymes. Body iron is concentrated in the storage forms, ferritin and hemosiderin, in bone marrow, liver, and spleen. Body iron stores can usually be estimated from the amount of ferritin protein in serum. Transferrin protein in the blood transports and delivers iron to cells.

Deficiencies. Severe iron deficiency results in anemia with small, pale, red blood cells that have a low hemoglobin concentration. Iron deficiency anemia in pregnancy increases the risk of premature and low birth weight babies. In young children, iron deficiency is associated with behavioural abnormalities (such as reduced attention span), and reduced cognitive performance that may not be fully reversible by iron replacement. In adults, severe iron deficiency anemia impairs physical work capacity. In the US, iron deficiency anemia is relatively rare, but affects 5 per cent of women 20 - 49 years old. Moderate iron deficiency without anemia is most common in 1 - 2 year-old children (9 per cent), and females 12 - 49 years old (9 - 11 per cent), reflecting rapid growth or menstrual iron loss, and is less common in other groups.

Dietary recommendations. The 1989 Recommended Dietary Allowance (RDA) for iron is 6 mg for infants through 6 months of age; 10 mg for older infants and children through 10 years old, men 18 years and older, and women over 50 years; 12 mg for 11-18 year-old males; 15 mg for 11-50 year-old females, including nursing mothers; and 30 mg (a recommendation which requires supplementation) during pregnancy. The 1989 - 91 USDA Food Consumption Survey indicates that average diets meet or exceed the RDA for all groups except 1-2 year-old children (91 per cent of RDA) and women ages 12-49 years (75-80 per cent of RDA). Iron supplements are not needed by most people and, because of potential adverse effects of excessive iron, should not be taken by adult men or postmenopausal women without demonstrable need.

Food sources. In the US, grain products are a principal source of dietary iron, followed by meat, poultry and fish, then vegetables, then legumes, nuts, and soy. Red meat is a rich source of iron that is well absorbed. Heme iron (about 40 per cent of the iron in meat, poultry, or fish, and 7-12 per cent of the iron in US diets) is 15-45 per cent absorbed, depending on iron stores (persons with low iron stores compensate by absorbing more iron). Nonheme iron, the remaining majority of dietary iron, is 1-15 per cent absorbed, depending on iron stores and on absorption enhancers (e.g., ascorbic acid, an unidentified factor in meat, poultry and fish) or inhibitors (e.g., phytic acid in whole grains and legumes, polyphenols in tea, coffee, or red wine, calcium in dairy products or supplements) eaten concurrently. In the US refined grain products are enriched routinely with iron. Iron-fortified formula or cereals are useful in preventing iron deficiency in infants.

Toxicity. Iron supplements intended for other household members are the most common cause of pediatric poisoning deaths in the US. In populations of European origin, approximately 1 in 300 people have hemochromatosis, a genetic abnormality of excessive iron stores. Ten percent of these populations carry a gene (are heterozygous) for hemochromatosis. Researchers are testing hypotheses that high iron stores may increase the risk of chronic diseases, such as cancer and h eart disease, through oxidative mechanisms.

Lipids

Lipids are defined as biological compounds soluble in organic solvents. The major categories are fatty acids, triacylglycerols (triglycerides), phospholipids, glycolipids (sphingolipids), sterols (such as cholesterol), and other iso-prenoids, fat-soluble vitamins, and waxes—each of which are composed of numerous subspecies. There are more than 1,000 different lipid species.

The term "fat" refers to triacylglycerols, which are composed of three fatty acid molecules attached to a glycerol backbone. The energy equivalent of fat is approximately 9 Calories per gram, which is more than twice the number for an equal weight of carbohydrate or protein. Triacylglycerols are stored primarily in adipocytes (fat cells). Triaglycerols (and other lipids) are transported in circulation as part of lipoproteins (lipids plus protein). The different types are: chylomicrons, very-low-density lipoproteins (VLDL), low-density lipoproteins (LDL), and high-density lipoproteins (HDL).

Lipids serve a variety of functions. Triacylglycerols are used for energy storage and insulation. Phospholipids, glycolipids and cholesterol are key building blocks of membranes and lipoproteins; they can also be converted to other highly bioactive compounds (such as platelet-derived growth factor, prostaglandins, diacylglycerols, ceramides, and steroid hormones) that participate in cell signaling. Cholesterol is converted to bile acids, which help emulsify food for digestion. Fat-soluble vitamins are involved in vision and cell regulation (A), calcium utilization (D), coagulation (K) and protection of membranes from oxidative damage (E and carotenoids).

Deficiencies. Only a few classes of lipids are required in the diet. These are the "essential" fatty acids (linoleic acid and alpha-linolenic acid), fat-soluble vitamins (vitamins A, D, E and K), and a number of other lipids that are mostly required under special circumstances, such as early in life or when digestion and utilization are not functioning fully.

Clinical uses. Enteral and parenteral formulations often contain lipids as sources of energy and essential fatty acids; supplements rich in unsaturated fatty acids (fish oils) have been used in treating atherosclerosis. Both are conducted under professional care.

Diet recommendations. The 1995 Dietary Guidelines for Americans recommends that intake of total fat be limited to no more than 30 percent of total calories by choosing lower fat options and increasing the amount and variety of grain products, fruits, and vegetables. Selection of foods based on the Food

Pyramid also reduces intake of saturated fat and cholesterol. Overall caloric intake should be matched to one's caloric needs combined with physical activity to maintain overall fitness. The limitation of fat percentage does not apply to infants and toddlers below the age of 2 years, but after that age, children should gradually adopt a diet that contains no more than 30 percent of calories from fat by about 5 years of age.

Toxicity. The major problem of lipid excess is the growing problem of overweight and obesity. This concern has been addressed in the Dietary Guidelines. Toxicity is also seen if vitamin A or D are consumed in excess of the Recommended Dietary Allowance (RDA).

Magnesium

Magnesium is the fourth most abundant cation in the body, with 60% in the bone and 40 per cent distributed equally between muscle and non-muscular soft tissue. Only 1 per cent of magnesium is extracellular. Magnesium has an important role in at least 300 fundamental enzymatic reactions, including the transfer of phosphate groups, the acylation of coenzyme A in the initiation of fatty acid oxidation, and the hydrolysis of phosphate and pyrophosphate. In addition, it functions in the activation of amino acids and synthesis and degradation of DNA and has a key role in neurotransmission and immune function. Magnesium acts as a calcium antagonist and interacts with nutrients, such as potassium, vitamin B6, and boron.

Deficiencies. Because the kidneys are extremely efficient in maintaining homeostasis of magnesium, a primary deficiency in healthy individuals is uncommon. Symptomatic deficiency is often observed in the presence of a predisposing disease state, such as severe malabsorption, chronic alcoholism, renal dysfunction, hyperparathyroidism, or the use of certain medications. Clinical manifestations of deficiency are related to its role as a cofactor in enzymatic reactions and in regulating neurotransmitters. Hypertension, arrhythmias, neuromuscular manifestations, and personality changes occur during deficiency.

Clinical uses. Accepted clinical uses of magnesium include the treatment of tachycardia and electrolyte depletion. It is also used for the management of premature labor, and for the prophylaxis and treatment of seizures in toxemia of pregnancy and hypomagnesemia associated with such conditions as alcoholism, Crohn's disease and hyperthyroidism. Magnesium is an active ingredient in antacids and laxatives.

Diet recommendations. The 1997 Dietary Reference Intakes (DRIs) and the Tolerable Upper Limits (ULs) for magnesium from the Food and Nutrition Board, National Academy of Sciences have been published. The DRIs, according to age and sex, are as follows: Infants 0-6 months, 30 mg and 7-12 months, 75 mg; ages 1-3 years, 80 mg; 4-8 years, 130 mg; 9-13 years, 240 mg; males 14-18 years, 410 mg; males 19-30 years, 400 mg; males >30 years, 420 mg; females 14-18 years, 360 mg; females 19-30 years, 310 mg; and females >30 years, 320 mg. Since no adverse effects from naturally occurring magnesium in foods have been observed, the UL applies only to supplements and magnesium for pharmacological purposes. The ULs are as follows: 1-3 years, 65 mg; 4-8 years, 110 mg; and 9 years and above, 350 mg.

Food sources. Good dietary sources of magnesium include legumes, whole grain cereals, nuts, dark green vegetables, and cocoa. Hard water and mineral water may be important sources of magnesium.

Niacin

Niacin (nicotinic acid or nicotinamide) is essential in the form of the coenzymes NAD and NADP in which the nicotinamide moiety acts as electron acceptor or hydrogen donor in many biological redox reactions. NAD functions as an electron carrier for intracellular respiration as well as a codehydrogenase with enzymes involved in the oxidation of fuel molecules. NADP functions as a hydrogen donor in reductive biosyntheses such as in fatty acid and steroid syntheses and, like NAD, as a co-dehydrogenase. NAD, in its only non-redox role, is the substrate for three classes of enzymes that transfer ADP-ribose units to proteins involved in DNA processing, cell differentiation, and cellular calcium mobilization.

Nicotinic acid and nicotinamide are rapidly absorbed from the stomach or the intestine. Nicotinamide, the major form in the bloodstream, arises from enzymatic hydrolysis of NAD(P) in the intestinal mucosa and liver, and is transported to tissues that synthesize their own NAD as needed. Niacin and NAD are biosynthesized from dietary tryptophan via the kynurenine pathway and quinolinic acid. Excess niacin is excreted in the urine primarily as Nl-methylnicotinamide and Nl-methyl-2-pyridone-5-carboxamide.

Deficiencies. Pellagra, the classic niacin deficiency disease, is characterized by bilateral dermatitis, diarrhea, and dementia. Often associated with a largely cereal diet such as maize or sorghum, the disease is now rarely seen in industrialized countries but still appears in India, China, and Africa. Pellagra often is associated with other micronutrient deficiencies and may develop also in cases of disturbed tryptophan metabolism (carcinoid syndrome, Hartnup's).

Diet recommendations. The RDA is expressed in mg niacin equivalents (NE) in which 1 mg NE = 1 mg niacin or 60 mg tryptophan. For individuals above 13 years of age, the 1998 RDA is 16 mg/d for males and 14 mg/d for females, with an additional allowance of 4 mg/d during pregnancy and 3 mg/d during lactation. The RDAs range from 6-12 mg/d for children 1-13 years and 2-3 mg/d for infants to one year.

Food sources. Niacin is widely distributed in plant and animal foods, mainly as the pyridine nucleotides NAD and NADP. Good sources are yeast, meats including liver, cereals, legumes, seeds, milk, green leafy vegetables, and fish.

Clinical uses. Nicotinic acid (but not nicotinamide) given as a drug in doses of 1.5-3 g/d improves the blood cholesterol profile. Nicotinamide acts as a tumor-specific radiosensitizer, possibly due to its effect on vasorelaxation and increased tumor oxygenation.

Toxicity. Large doses of nicotinic acid given to lower cholesterol may produce flushing of the skin, hyperuricemia, and hepatic abnormalities. These effects are reversed if the drug is reduced in amount or discontinued. The 1998 Tolerable Upper Intake Level (UL) of niacin, based on flushing produced by nicotinic acid, is 35 mg/d for adults.

Phosphorus

Phosphorus (P) is an essential mineral that is found in all cells within the body. The body of the human adult contains about 400-500 g. The greatest amount of body phosphorus can be found primarily in bone (85 per cent) and muscle (14 per cent). Phosphorus is primarily found as phosphate (PO_4^{2-}). The major building blocks of biology are covalent molecules comprising proteins, polysaccharides, and nucleic acids. The nucleic acids deoxyribonucleic acid (DNA) and ribonucleic acid (RNA) are polymers based on phosphate ester monomers. The high-energy phosphate bond of ATP is the major energy currency of living organisms. Cell membranes are composed largely of phospholipids. The inorganic constituents of bone are primarily a calcium phosphate salt called hydroxyapatite. A variety of enzymatic activities are controlled by alternate phosphorylation and dephosphorylation of proteins. The metabolism of all major metabolic substrates depends on the functioning of phosphorus as a cofactor in a variety of enzymes and as the principal reservoir for metabolic energy.

Deficiencies. Dietary phosphorus absorption is about 60-70 per cent; any excess absorbed is readily excreted in the urine. Since renal conservation of phosphorus occurs quite efficiently on low phosphorus diets, a deficiency rarely occurs in a healthy population. However, various disease states or conditions (e.g., gastrointestinal malabsorption, diabetes mellitus, renal tubular dysfunction, antacid abuse, and premature birth) can be associated with low blood phosphorus levels (i.e., hypophosphatemia) and depleted phosphorus stores.

Diet recommendations. New recommendations for dietary phosphorus include a value, the Recommended Dietary Allowance (RDA), which an individual should aim to meet, and a value, the Tolerable Upper Level (UL), which should not be exceeded. Intakes between the RDA and the UL ensure that serum phosphorus levels will be maintained in the normal range. Values for infants are called Adequate Intake (AI) levels, and are based on a significant portion of intake being from breast milk. It should also be noted that there are no additional requirements for P during pregnancy or lactation. The Recommended intake levels for P (mg per day) are set based on life stage groups. For infants 0 to 6, and 6 to 12 months, the RDA is 100 and 275 mg, respectively. No UL has been set for these ages as supplementation would be unlikely. For children 1 to 3 and 4 to 8 years, the RDA is 460 and 500, respectively, and the UL is 3000 mg. For youth 9 to 18 years, the RDA is 1250 mg, which indicates the higher need for phosphorus during the adolescent growth spurt; the UL for youth is 4000 mg. Adults 19 years and older have an RDA of 700 mg. The UL is 4000 mg up to age 70, then declines to 3000 mg after age 70 years.

Food Sources. Phosphorus is found widely distributed in foodstuffs. In the United States, the average daily intake is about 1600 mg for males and 1000 mg for females. In general, food sources rich in protein (milk, meat, eggs, legumes and grains) are also high in phosphorus. The relative contributions of food groups to phosphorus intake are: 60 per cent from milk, meat, poultry, fish, and eggs; 20 per cent from cereals and legumes; 10 per cent from fruits and fruit juices; 4 per cent from alcoholic beverages; and 3 per cent from soft drinks and other beverages.

Toxicity. A diet containing a 2:1 dietary ratio of phosphorus to calcium can cause low blood calcium (hypocalcemia) and secondary hyperparathyroidism with excess bone resorption and bone loss in animals. Human breast milk, with a lower phosphorus content than cow milk, is considered better suited to the needs of the infant. For older ages, typical diets in the United States frequently exceed the recommended ratio; however, these diets are not believed to be harmful unless calcium intake is also very low. As intake of phosphorus rises, so does serum phosphorus. Elevated serum phosphorus levels (hyperphosphatemia) can occur in patients with renal failure due to a poor ability to excrete phosphorus in the urine. As indicated by UL values, intake of phosphorus exceeding 3 to 4 grams may be harmful in healthy individuals.

Potassium

Potassium (K) in the form of K^+ is the most essential cation of the cells. Its high intracellular concentration is regulated by the cell membrane through the sodium-potassium pump. Most of the total body potassium is found in muscle tissue. Total body potassium has been used as a measure of lean body mass, of muscle mass, or (more accurately) of cell mass. Because of its association with the metabolizing, oxygen-consuming portion of the body, a decline in total body potassium is usually interpreted as a loss of muscle mass due to a catabolic condition. Potassium exists in nature in three isotopes: ^{39}K (93.26 per cent), ^{40}K (0.0117 per cent) and ^{41}K (6.73 per cent). ^{40}K is radioactive and responsible for most of the naturally occurring internal radioactivity in the body. This property enables investigators to monitor total body potassium values as a function of age and disease.

Deficiencies. With the exception of starvation, low or declining total body potassium is not a result of insufficient dietary intake but the outcome of a catabolic, protein wasting condition which reduces the total cell mass of the body. Hypokalemia (low serum K) is the result of excessive loss of K in the urine, usually as a result of use of diuretic agents to treat hypertension. Hypokalemia may result in cardiac failure.

Dietary recommendations. The Estimated Minimum Requirement for potassium for adolescents and adults is 2000 mg or 50 mEq/day. The usual dietary intake for adults is about 100 mEq/day. For hypertension patients using diuretic medications, it is recommended often to supplement their diet with orange juice, bananas and vegetables which contain high amounts of potassium. Increased potassium intake helps maintain normal plasma levels. However, the blood level of potassium (which is sensitive to diet) is not indicative of total body potassium which is an index of cell mass and muscle.

Food sources. Most foods contain potassium. The best food sources are fruits, vegetables and juices; potassium also is present in meats and cereals. There is no known food supplement which would directly increase total body potassium by compensating for a dietary potassium deficiency.

Toxicity. The fraction of potassium which is present outside the cells plays an active role in the propagation of electrical signals between neurons, skeletal muscle function and regulation of blood pressure. Urinary excretion protects against the accumulation of high levels of potassium. However, acute hyperkalemia can be lethal by causing cardiac arrest.

Protein

Proteins are polymers of amino acids that contain the elements carbon, hydrogen, oxygen, nitrogen and sulfur. Particular emphasis is given to the indispensable amino acids, i.e., those that must be in the food supply because they either cannot be synthesized in the body or they cannot be synthesized in adequate quantity to meet the needs for optimal rates of growth in children. The indispensable amino acids are: lysine, methionine, threonine, tryptophan, leucine, isoleucine, valine, phenylalanine, arginine and histidine. A dietary supply of arginine is not required by adults. The amino acids supplied from dietary protein are needed for synthesis of body proteins in muscle, organs, bone and skin, and for synthesis of enzymes, certain hormones, antibodies and a host of specialized products.

Deficiencies. Deficiencies of protein or of one or more of the indispensable amino acids will lead to reduced growth in children or loss of muscle mass in adults. Susceptibility to disease will be increased, and in extreme cases, death may result. Protein-energy malnutrition is often described in its two extreme forms: marasmus which is a generalized wasting due to a deficiency of both protein and energy, and kwashiorkor which is characterized by edema and a deficiency of both protein quantity and quality (i.e., poor pattern of indispensable amino acids).

Food sources. Virtually all unprocessed foods contain protein, and the protein of these foods is characterized by the quantity and ratio of indispensable amino acids (protein quality) contained therein. Animal proteins (meat, milk, eggs) are considered to be excellent in both protein quantity and quality. Plant proteins vary in protein quantity and quality. Members of the bean family: soybeans, kidney beans, navy beans, and lima beans are rich in protein, and the protein quality is quite good as well. Split peas and lentils fall into the same category. Potatoes are rich in protein quality but not in quantity. Breads, cereals, fruits and most leaf and stem vegetables are not considered good sources of high-quality protein. Combining certain foods together (e.g. beans with corn) results in a complementary effect in which the protein quality of the combination is superior to either food consumed alone.

Diet recommendations. Recommended dietary allowances attempt to make allowances for protein quality differences in foods typically consumed by the US population. Surveys have indicated that animal-source proteins contribute 65 per cent of the daily protein ingested by humans in the US. Protein requirements increase with advancing age up to 50 years (63 g/day for males, 50 g/day for females) and then plateau. Children of both sexes between 7 and 10 years of age are estimated to require 28 g/day. Additional protein is needed for pregnancy (+10 g/day) and lactation (+15 g/day). Dietary surveys indicate that adult Americans consume more-than-adequate amounts of protein (men, 90 g; women 70 g).

Riboflavin

Riboflavin (vitamin B-2) is chemically known as 7, 8-dimethyl-10 (1'-D-ribityl) isoalloxazine. In tissues there is a broad distribution of flavin but little is present as free riboflavin. The majority is found in flavocoenzymes [mainly flavin adenine dinucleotide (FAD)] and lesser amounts are in a mononucleotide [riboflavin-5'-phosphate (FMN)]. Levels of flavin range from a few μg/g wet weight in skeletal muscle and intestine, and up to 30 to 35 μg/g in liver and kidney. Flavocoenzymes are largely non-covalently associated within diverse flavoproteins, but some exist as 8-a-linked FAD.

As the catalytically operating moiety within bound flavocoenzymes, riboflavin participates in oxidation-reduction reactions in numerous metabolic pathways and in energy production via the respiratory chain. Flavoproteins participate in both one- and two-electron transfers. They operate in pyridine nucleotide-dependent and independent and independent dehydrogenations, reactions with sulfur-containing compounds, hydroxylation, oxidative decarboxylations, deoxygenations, and reduction of oxygen to hydrogen peroxide following abstraction of hydrogen from substrates.

Deficiencies. Ariboflavinosis is characterized by weakness, sore throat, hyperemia and edema of the pharyngeal and oral mucous membranes, cheilosis, angular stomatitis, glossitis, seborrheic dermatitis, corneal vascularization, and normochromic, normocytic anemia associated with pure red cell hypoplasia of the bone marrow.

Clinical uses. Riboflavin is used therapeutically to ameliorate ariboflavinosis resulting from diverse causes such as inadequate dietary intake, decreased assimilation, rare genetic defects in the formation of specific flavoproteins, hormonal disorders and after use of certain drugs. Also, riboflavin supplements are provided during treatment of neonatal jaundice with phototherapy. The side chain of the vitamin is photochemically destroyed as it is involved in the photosensitized oxidation of bilirubin to more polar excretable compounds.

Diet recommendations. Suggested amounts range from an Adequate Intake of 0.3 mg/day for early infants to RDAs of 1.1 mg/day for women and 1/3 mg/day for men. An additional 0.3 mg/day is recommended during pregnancy and 0.4 mg/day for lactation.

Food sources. Small amounts of riboflavin, occurring largely as digestible coenzymes, are present in most plant and animal tissues. Especially good sources are milk, eggs, enriched cereals and grains, ice cream, liver, some lean meats, and green vegetables such as broccoli. As much as a third of North American intake is attributed to milk and other dairy products.

Toxicity. The limited capacity to absorb orally administered riboflavin precludes its potential for harm. Riboflavin intake of many times the RDA is without demonstrable toxicity. Nevertheless, the photosensitizing properties of riboflavin raise the possibility of some theoretical, potential risks.

Sodium

Sodium (Na) is the predominant cation in extracellular fluid and its concentration is under tight homeostatic control. Excess dietary sodium is excreted in the urine. The mineral is very efficiently reabsorbed by the kidney when intakes are low or losses are excessive. Sodium acts in consort with potassium, the chief cation of intracellular fluid, to maintain proper body water distribution and blood pressure. Sodium also is important in maintaining the proper acid-base balance and in the transmission of nerve impulses.

Deficiencies. Persons who experience pronounced losses of sodium through diarrhea, heavy perspiration or inability of the kidney to reabsorb it may experience decreased blood volume and a fall in blood pressure that could result in shock.

Diet recommendations. The Estimated Minimum Requirement of Healthy Persons for sodium from the National Academy of Sciences ranges from 120 mg/day for infants to 500 mg/day for adults and children >10 years. Recommendations for the maximum amount of sodium that can be incorporated into a healthy diet range from 2,400 to 3,000 mg/day or 6 to 7.5 grams of table salt/day. Individuals with hypertension should see their physician to determine if a sodium-restricted diet is appropriate for them.

The usual dietary intake of sodium in the US and other populations where salt is readily available ranges from about 2,300 to 4,500 mg/day. Mean sodium intake for the entire US population is 3,280 mg Na or 8.2 grams salt /day; however, discretionary salt intake is not included. Intake of discretionary salt, that added during cooking and at the table, averages 2.7 g/day according to the National Health and Nutrition Examination Survey. A diet based on Asian foods, such as those seasoned with soy sauce and monosodium glutamate, may contain the equivalent of 30 to 40 grams salt/day.

The appropriateness of current recommendations for the general healthy population to reduce sodium intake has been a matter of debate in the scientific community. Public health scientists generally support the population-wide approach, while many clinically- or laboratory-oriented scientists are unconvinced that the population approach has sufficient benefit to offset the potential burden—to either consumers or industry— associated with sodium reduction. In addition, although sodium reduction to the levels recommended is presumed to be safe for healthy adults, the debate about this issue has been fueled by assertions that sodium reduction might have adverse effects on health. These assertions about adverse effects appear unwarranted.

Food sources. Sodium added to processed foods accounts for the majority of sodium (75 per cent) in the US diet. The remainder comes from discretionary salt (15 per cent) and the sodium that occurs naturally in foods (10 per cent). A substantial portion of sodium in foods is hidden in the sense that it occurs in foods that are moderate in sodium content and that are not thought of as salty foods, e.g:, processed grain and cereal products, but which are consumed regularly. Other contributors to high sodium intake are foods with high amounts of salt. High amounts of salt are found in table salt and soy sauce, followed by foods in brine such as pickles, olives and sauerkraut. Salty or smoked meats and fish, salted snack foods, bouillon cubes, bottled sauces, processed cheeses, and canned and instant soups also contain significant levels of sodium.

Toxicity. Acute toxicity results in edema and hypertension and can cause death in an infant because of limited excretory ability of the immature kidney. However, sodium is generally nontoxic for healthy adult individuals because it is excreted readily in the urine. High salt intakes have been correlated with hypertension. Meta analyses suggest that a reduction in sodium intake of 2,300/day would lower systolic blood pressure by about 5-6 mm Hg and diastolic pressure by 1-2 mm Hg among hypertensives, who comprise a sizeable proportion of the US adult population. In addition, many who are not yet hypertensive respond to sodium reduction, particularly those whose blood pressure is in the high normal range. The expected impact of a similar reduction among the normotensive segment of the population is considerably smaller (1-2 mm Hg systolic and 0-1 mm Hg diastolic on average). Sodium reduction among normotensives is primarily designed to effect a downward shift in the average blood pressure in the population, with consequent impact in preventing a large number of cardiovascular disease deaths. High sodium intake or intake of highly salted foods may also be related to asthma, to urinary calcium losses, and to gastric cancer.

Thiamin

Thiamin (vitamin B-1) is a water-soluble substance, consisting of thiazole and pyrimidine rings joined by a methylene bridge. Thiamin is found in high concentrations in skeletal muscle, the heart, liver, kidneys and brain. The total amount in an adult is about 30 mg and the biologic half-life in the body is about 15 days. It is not surprising that a state of severe depletion can be seen in patients on a strict thiamin-deficient diet in 18 days. Similarly, the rate of flux of thiamin across the blood-brain barrier in rats is equivalent to the turnover in brain, indicating no spare thiamin capacity for the brain.

Thiamin diphosphate (ThDP) is the active form of thiamin. ThDP serves as a cofactor for several enzymes involved in carbohydrate catabolism, including pyruvate dehydrogenase, transketolase, and a-ketoglutarate, and for the branched-chain a-keto acid dehydrogenase complex that is involved in amino acid catabolism. The former enzymes play crucial roles in the tricarboxylic acid cycle and the pentose phosphate pathway. They are important in the biosynthesis of a number of cell constituents, including the neurotransmitters acetylcholine and gamma-aminobutyric acid (GABA), and in the production of reducing equivalents (NADPH) for biosyntheses and pentoses for nucleic acid synthesis. Because of its involvement in the synthesis of precursors of DNA, thiamin utilization is increased in tumors. Limiting thiamin can inhibit tumor cell proliferation. A neurochemical role for thiamin triphosphate (ThTP) has been postulated; ThTP is localized to neuronal cells and is implicated in neuronal conduction.

Thiamin uptake by the small intestines and by cells within various organs is mediated at physiological concentrations by a saturable, high affinity transport system. The requirement for cellular energy (ATP) for thiamin uptake is a secondary event and results from the rapid diphosphorylation of imported thiamin by thiamin diphosphokinase. Alcohol affects various aspects of thiamin transport/uptake, and these effects may contribute to the prevalence of thiamin deficiency in alcoholics. Alcohol also reduces cellular thiamin diphosphokinase activity.

Deficiencies. The major manifestations of thiamin deficiency in humans involve the cardiovascular (wet beriberi) and nervous (dry beriberi, or neuropathy and/or Wernicke-Korsakoff syndrome) systems. Common findings in beriberi heart disease include peripheral vasodilation, biventricular myocardial failure, and sodium and water retention resulting in high-output state, edema, and potentially acute fulminant cardiovascular collapse (soshin beriberi). Administration of thiamin rapidly restores peripheral vascular resistance, but improvement in myocardial function may be delayed. The predominant features of cerebral beriberi are confusion, disordered ocular motility, ataxia of gait, and neuropathy. Treatment with thiamin can rapidly reverse some of these acute signs while leaving significant clinical sequelae including memory and other cognitive deficits and residual neurologic signs (called Korsakoff's syndrome, or the chronic phase of Wernicke-Korsakoff syndrome) with characteristic neuropathologic findings. Recently, amyloid-precursor protein-like immunoreactivity, similar to findings in Alzheimer's patients, have been demonstrated in the brains of thiamin deficient rats consistent with earlier suggestions of a relationship between thiamin deficiency and Alzheimer's disease.

Additionally, a number of inborn errors of metabolism have been described in which clinical improvements can be documented following administration of pharmacological doses of thiamin, including thiamin-responsive megaloblastic anemia (TRMA), lactic acidosis, branched chain ketoaciduria, and intermittent cerebellar ataxia. TRMA results from a lack of the saturable, high affinity thiamin transport system, and ketoaciduria results from defects in the branch-chain a-keto acid dehydrogenase.

Diet recommendations. The Recommended Dietary Allowance is as follows: 0-5 month infants, 0.2 mg/day; 6 to 11 months, 0.3 mg/day; 1-3 years of age, 0.5 mg/day; 4-8 years, 0.6 mg/day; 9-13 years, 0.9 mg/day; males 14 years old and older, 1.2 mg/day; females 14-18 years of age, 1.0 mg/day; and females 19 years and older, 1.1 mg/day. During pregnancy, the RDA is increased to 1.4 mg/day, and during lactation, 1.5 mg/day. The RDAs are based on the Dietary Reference Intakes of the National Academy of Sciences.

Food sources. Thiamin is present in many dietary products, but is found in large amounts in lean pork, legumes and yeast. Whole grain products, breads and cereals are the major dietary contributors.

Clinical uses. Therapy in deficiency consists of parenteral administration of thiamin (intramuscular or intravenous) as 50-100 mg/day for 7-14 days, followed by oral therapy. In clinical disorders related to thiamin deficiency, therapy is urgent and should bypass the intestinal tract. More moderate doses may be prudent for cancer patients in need of nourishment.

Toxicity. There is no toxicity with oral thiamin. There are only a few reports of toxic reactions to intravenous thiamin, resulting mainly in an anaphylactic reaction.

Vitamin A

The chemical name of vitamin A is retinol [3, 7-dimethyl-9-(2,6,6, trimethyl-1-cyclohexen-1-yl)-2,4,6,8-natetraen-1-ol]. Retinol is also found as retynyl (vitamin A) esters such as retinyl acetate and retinyl palmitate. The major storage site of vitamin A in the body is in the liver, primarily in the form of retinyl esters.

The best known function of vitamin A is in vision, where it participates (as the metabolite retinal) in the visual cycle. However, in the chemical form retinoic acid, vitamin A plays an important role in control of gene expression. This function maintains differentiation of epithelial cells such as skin, lung, and intestinal tissue. Retinoic acid can be formed from retinol in the body, and shows strong biological activity in some functions but not in vision.

Deficiencies. Night blindness is one of the early signs of vitamin A deficiency, because of the role of vitamin A in vision. Bacterial invasion and permanent scarring of the cornea of the eye (xerophthalmia) is a symptom of more profound deficiency, but this is due to a different mechanism, the lack of vitamin A for control of gene expression. Profound vitamin A deficiency also results in altered appearance and function of skin, lung, and intestinal tissues. Children are most at risk of vitamin A deficiency because they have not yet developed adequate vitamin A stores. It has been estimated that 0.5 million children in the world become blind each year, 70 per cent of these due to vitamin A deficiency. Over half of these blind children die from malnutrition and associated illnesses.

Diet recommendations. For adult human males, the Recommended Dietary Allowance (RDA) is 1000 ug Retinyl Equivalents (RE)/d; for adult females, 800 ug RE.

Food sources. The RDA can be met by consuming dietary preformed vitamin A (retinyl esters) from liver, eggs and fortified foods, and provitamin A carotenoids such as beta-carotene, which are found in green leafy vegetables as well as in orange and red fruits and vegetables.

Clinical uses. Synthetic retinoids such as 13-cis retinoic acid (trade name Accutane, also known as isotretinoin) are used to treat acne and skin wrinkling. Other derivatives, such as 4-hydroxyphenylretinamide (4-HPR, Fenretinide), are used to treat breast cancer. No one should consume vitamin A in quantities exceeding the RDA without a doctor's advice because of the dangers of toxicity.

Toxicity. Acute intake of extremely high doses of vitamin A (>200 mg RE in adult humans) can cause nausea, vomiting, headache, and increased cerebrospinal pressure. Symptoms are generally transient. Chronic high intakes (e.g., >10x RDA) can cause hair loss, bone and muscle pain, headache, liver damage, and increased blood lipid concentrations. A particular danger in pregnant women is teratogenesis (birth defects). On the other hand, carotenoids as a source of vitamin A are not toxic, even with very high intakes.

Vitamin B-12

Vitamin B-12 (cobalamin), stored in the liver, is a cofactor for two coenzymes. Methyl-cobalamin catalyzes methyl group transfer from a folic acid cofactor to form methionine; the unmethylated folate cofactor then participates in single carbon reactions for nucleic acid synthesis. Thus some B-12 and folic deficiency symptoms are similar. The B-12 coenzyme deoxyadenosylcobalamin catalyzes amino acid and fatty acid breakdown.

Deficiencies. Stages of deficiency symptoms include Stage I (early deficiency), lower serum holoTC II (<60 pg/mL); Stage II, lower serum vitamin B-12 (<300 pg/mL) and holoTC II (<40 pg/mL); Stage III, serum B-12 <200 and holoTC II <40 pg/mL, neutrophil hypersegmentation, elevated serum and urinary methylmalonic acid and homocysteine; and Stage IV (severest deficiency), also megaloblastic, macrocytic anemia. Around Stage III (before anemia), potentially irreversible demyelination of spinal cord, brain, and optic and peripheral nerves produces peripheral neuropathy progressing to subacute combined degeneration. Dementia, poor attention span, and depression may be early symptoms.

The stomach secretes intrinsic factor that binds B-12 and mediates its absorption at receptor sites in the ileum. Inadequate intrinsic factor secretion occurs in pernicious anemia, an autoimmune disease. In the elderly, atrophic gastritis is commonly associated with B-12 malabsorption and deficiency. Because the absorbed vitamin is secreted in bile and subsequently reabsorbed, deficiency symptoms can take 20 years to develop from low intakes, e.g., in strict vegetarians. However, in malabsorption, deficiency occurs in months or a few years because absorption from both the diet and enterohepatic circulation is impaired.

Diet recommendations. The Recommended Daily Allowances (RDAs) are (µg/day): 0.3 at age 0-6 months, 0.5 for 6-12 months, 0.7 for 1-3 years, 1.0 for 4-6 years, 1.4 for 7-10 years, 2.0 for adolescents and adults, 2.2 in pregnancy and 2.6 in lactation. Usual intakes are about 4-8 µg/d. Pregnant, lactating, and long-term strict vegetarians should take supplements providing the RDA.

Food sources. Vitamin B-12 is found only in animal products. Excellent sources (>10 µg/100g) include organ meats and bivalve mollusks such as clams and oysters. Moderate amounts (1-10 µg/100g) are contained in egg yolks, muscle meats and poultry, fish, fermented cheeses and dry milk. Milk and milk products contain <1 µg/100g. There is no human-active form of B-12 in algae such as nori and spirulina; the forms are all analogues.

Toxicity. No toxic effects have been reported when up to 100 µg/day are consumed. Intramuscular injections of 100 µg are usually given once/month to individuals who cannot absorb the vitamin through their intestine, because of pernicious anemia or other problems.

Vitamin B-6

The chemical name of vitamin B_6 is pyridoxine hydrochloride; 2-methyl-3-hydroxy-4,5-bis (hydroxy-methyl) pyridine. Other forms of vitamin B_6 include pyridoxal, and pyridoxamine. In the body all three of these compounds can be phosphorylated. About 70-80 per cent of the vitamin B_6 in the body is located in muscle bound to glycogen phosphorylase, an enzyme involved in releasing glucose from glycogen. About 10 per cent is located in the liver; the remainder is distributed among the other tissues.

B_6 is one of the most versatile enzyme cofactors. It is involved in breaking more types of chemical bonds than most cofactors. It is listed in Enzyme Nomenclature as a component of approximately 120 enzymes including at least one entry in 5 of the 6 major enzyme classes. Pyridoxal phosphate is a cofactor in the metabolism of amino acids and neurotransmitters and in the breakdown of glycogen. Pyridoxal phosphate can bind to steroid hormone receptors and may have a role in regulating steroid hormone action. Pyridoxal phosphate can be converted to pyridoxamine phosphate which can also serve as an enzyme cofactor. 4-pyridoxic acid is the major excretory product.

Deficiencies. Alterations in the function of the nervous system evidenced by electroencephalography are among the earliest symptoms of vitamin B-6 deficiency. Severe deficiency may produce seizures, dermatitis, glossitis, cheilosis, angular stomatitis and anemia. Frank deficiencies are rare, but subclinical deficiencies may exist, especially in women and the elderly.

Diet recommendations. Adequate Intakes (AI) have been set at 0.1 mg/d for infants up to 6 mo. and 0.3 mg/d for 6 mo. to 1 yr. Recommended Dietary Allowances (RDAs) (mg/d) for children have been set at 0.5 (1-3 yr.), 0.6 (4-8 yr.), and 1.0 (9-13 yr.). For men the RDAs (mg/d) are 1.3 (14-50 yr.) and 1.7 (51+ yr.). For women the RDAs (mg/d) are 1.2 (14 - 18 yrs.), 1.3 (19-50 yr.), 1.5 (51+ yr.), 1.9 during pregnancy, and 2.0 during lactation.

Food sources. White meats (poultry, fish, pork), bananas and whole grains are good sources of vitamin B_6.

Clinical uses. Pyridoxine-dependent seizures and some types of sideroblastic anemias respond to vitamin B_6 supplementation. Vitamin B_6 in conjunction with folate and vitamin B_{12} helps to lower plasma homocysteine, a risk factor for heart disease. Vitamin B_6 supplements may be required in conjunction with a number of drugs which have the side-effect of altering vitamin B_6 metabolism. Increased concentrations of pyridoxal phosphate in plasma are used as one of the criteria for diagnosing hypophosphatasia. Because vitamin B_6 metabolism is altered in a variety of disease states, there have been suggestions that vitamin B_6 supplements may be beneficial in many other conditions. However, convincing scientific support is not currently available.

Vitamin C

Vitamin C is also known as ascorbic acid, L-ascorbic acid, dehydroascorbic acid and the antiscorbutic vitamin. Chemically, it is called L-xyloascorbic acid and L-threo-hex-2-uronic acidy-lactone. The very highest concentrations of vitamin C are found in the adrenal and pituitary glands. High levels are also found in liver, leukocytes, brain, kidney and pancreas. Most of the vitamin C is found in liver and skeletal muscle because of their size relative to the rest of the body.

The best characterized function of vitamin C is in the synthesis of collagen connective tissue protein at the level of hydroxylation of prolyl and lysyl residues of procollagen. Vitamin C also plays important roles in the synthesis of neurotransmitters, steroid hormones, carnitine, conversion of cholesterol to bile acids, tyrosine degradation and metal ion metabolism. This vitamin also may enhance iron bioavailability. The role of ascorbic acid as a biological reducing agent may be linked to its prevention of degenerative diseases, such as cataracts, certain cancers and cardiovascular diseases.

Deficiencies. Severe ascorbic acid deficiency results in clinical scurvy which is characterized by swollen, bleeding gums, loosening of the teeth, capillary hemorrhaging, including bleeding into joints, tender and painful extremities, poor wound healing, weakness and fatigue, and psychological disturbances.

Clinical uses. The only established use of vitamin C is in the prevention and treatment of scurvy. Studies investigating possible effects on wound healing, blood pressure, colds and immune function have been epidemiological in nature or have often employed other antioxidants in addition to ascorbic acid. In most cases, the results have been unremarkable, conflicting or inconsistent, but research and interest continue in these areas.

Diet recommendations. The Recommended Dietary Allowance (RDA) for adults is 60 mg/day in the US, but may range from 30-75 mg/day in other Western countries. Intakes of 75-95 mg/day are recommended for pregnant and lactating women. The RDA is 35 mg/day in infants and 40 mg/day in children, ages 1-3 yr. About 10 mg/day is required to prevent scurvy. Increased intake of vitamin C is recommended for stress situations such as trauma, infection, strenuous exercise, or elevated environmental temperatures. The requirement in smokers may be 100 mg/day. Recent kinetic analyses suggest that intakes of 150-200 mg/day, but below 400 mg/day, obtained from the diet, may offer the most benefit in normal, healthy individuals.

Food sources. The best food sources of vitamin C are citrus fruits, berries, melons, tomatoes, potatoes, green peppers and leafy green vegetables. Vitamin C is sensitive to air, heat and water, so it can easily be destroyed by prolonged storage, overcooking and processing of foods.

Toxicity. Megadoses of vitamin C of 1000-2000 mg have commonly been associated with gastrointestinal disturbances (nausea, abdominal cramps and diarrhea). In general, megadoses of vitamin C should be avoided in individuals with a history of renal stones due to oxalate formation or hemochromatosis or other diseases related to excessive iron accumulation. Excess vitamin C may predispose premature infants to hemolytic anemia due to the fragility of their red blood cells. In healthy individuals, it appears that megadoses of up to 1000 mg/day of vitamin C are well tolerated and not associated with any consistent adverse effects. Concern of its pro-oxidant properties is stimulating renewed interest in its potential long-term toxicity.

Vitamin D

Vitamin D3 (cholecalciferol) and vitamin D2 (ergocalciferol) are stored in body fat. The vitamin D precursors produced in yeast and plants (ergosterol) and animals (7-dehydrocholesterol) are converted to vitamin D by exposure to ultraviolet light (290-315 nm). Vitamin D (either vitamin D2 or vitamin D3) is metabolized in the liver to 25-hydroxyvitamin D and then to 1, 25-dihydroxyvitamin D in the kidney. 1, 25-Dihydroxyvitamin D is considered to be the biologically functioning form of vitamin D. The major functions of vitamin D are to increase the efficiency of intestinal calcium absorption and to mobilize calcium stores from bone in order to maintain the serum calcium and phosphorus concentrations within the normal physiological range.

Deficiencies. In humans, deficiency symptoms include rickets in children, osteomalacia in adults, muscle weakness, bony deformities, neuromuscular irritability causing muscle spasms of the larynx (laryngospasm) and hands (carpopedal spasm), generalized convulsions and tetany.

Clinical uses. Vitamin D is useful for preventing and treating vitamin D-deficiency bone diseases (rickets in children and osteomalacia in adults). 25-Hydroxyvitamin D3 is useful for treating disorders, such as severe liver failure, in which vitamin D cannot be metabolized to 25-hydroxyvitamin D. The active form of vitamin D (1, 25-dihydroxyvitamin D3) and its analogs are useful for treating metabolic bone disorders due to inborn and acquired disorders in the metabolism of 1, 25-dihydroxyvitamin D2. These have recently been shown to also be valuable in treating the skin disease psoriasis.

Diet recommendations. The Institute of Medicine (IOM) for the National Academy of Sciences issued a report in August 1997 regarding new dietary guidelines for vitamin D. After careful review of the literature, the IOM concluded that it was not possible to determine a recommended dietary allowance (RDA) for vitamin D from the literature but rather to recommend an adequate intake (AI). Based on the available literature and assuming some exposure to sunlight, an AI for ages 0 - 50 years was set at 200 IU (5 ?g)/day. The IOM panel recognized that vitamin D insufficiency and deficiency are prevalent in adults over the age of 50 years and set the AI for adults 51 - 70 years as 400 IU (10 ?g)/day and for adults > 71 years, 600 IU (15 ?g)/day. There was no compelling data to increase the vitamin D requirement either during pregnancy or lactation. A Tolerable Upper Limit level for vitamin D for ages 0 - 12 months was set at a limit of 1,000 IU (25 ?g)/day. For older children and adults, including pregnant and lactating women, the UL was set at 2,000 IU (50 ?mg) day.

Food sources. Good food sources are milk properly fortified with vitamin D, fatty fish such as salmon and mackerel, cod liver oil, fish liver oil, some breads and cereals, and some egg yolks.

Toxicity. Excessive quantities of vitamin D (in excess of 5,000-10,000 IU/day) can cause hypercalcemia, hypercalciuria, kidney stones, and soft tissue calcifications.

Vitamin E

Vitamin E is an essential fat-soluble vitamin that includes eight naturally occurring compounds in two classes designated as tocopherols and tocotrienols. Each of these compounds exhibits different biological activities. d-?-Tocopherol has the highest biological activity and is the most widely available form of vitamin E in food. The other isomers (beta, delta, gamma), some of which are more abundant in a typical Western diet, are less biologically active than d-?-tocopherol. The commercially available synthetic forms of vitamin E are comprised of approximately an equal mixture of eight stereoisomeric forms of ?-tocopherol, usually in the esterified form such as acetate or succinate. For practical purposes, 1 International Unit (IU) of vitamin E represents 1 mg of the synthetic form, racemic a-tocopherol acetate, while the natural form of d-a-tocopherol has a biopotency of vitamin E equal to at least 1.49 IU, if not more. The most widely accepted biological function of vitamin E is its antioxidant properties. Vitamin E is the most effective chain-breaking, lipid-soluble antioxidant in biological membranes, where it contributes to membrane stability. It protects critical cellular structures against damage from oxygen free radicals and reactive products of lipid peroxidation.

Absorption of vitamin E is dependent upon the digestion and absorption of fat. Free tocopherols are absorbed by a non-saturable, passive process into the lymphatic circulation along with fat. About 45 per cent of an ordinary dose is absorbed into the lymph.

Deficiencies. The main signs of severe deficiency in animals are reproductive failure, nutritional "muscular dystrophy," hemolytic anemia, and neurological and immunological abnormalities. The last three processes also have been identified in humans. However, vitamin E deficiency occurs rarely in humans, having been reported in only two situations: premature infants with very low birth weight and patients who fail to absorb fat.

Diet recommendations. The Recommended Dietary Allowance (RDA) for vitamin E is based primarily on customary intakes from US food sources. The current RDA for males is 10 mg and 8 mg for females. However, the requirement for vitamin E increases with higher intakes of polyunsaturated fatty acids (PUFA). The recommended ratio of E/PUFA is 0.4 mg d-?-tocopherol per gram of PUFA. In defining the ideal intake, factors to consider are intake of other antioxidants, age, environmental pollutants, and physical activity.

Food sources. Vegetables and seed oils including soybean, safflower, and corn; sunflower seeds; nuts; whole grains; and wheat germ are the main sources of the tocopherols. Leafy vegetables also supply an appreciable amount of this nutrient. However, animal products and most fruits and vegetables are generally poor sources.

Toxicity. Vitamin E is relatively safe compared to the fat-soluble vitamins. Few side effects from high intakes of this vitamin have been reported, even at doses as high as 3200 mg daily. However, high vitamin E supplementation may be contraindicated when a coagulation defect is present due to vitamin K deficiency or in individuals receiving anticoagulant drugs.

Vitamin K

Vitamin K is a coenzyme for a microsomal enzyme that catalyzes the posttranslational conversion of specific glutamyl residues to gamma-carboxyglutamyl (Gla) residues in a small number of proteins. Several of the Gla-proteins are essential for blood clotting and its regulation (coagulation factors II, VII, IX, and X; proteins C, S and Z). Others have a role in the regulation of tissue mineralization (osteocalcin, matrix Gla protein) and cell proliferation (gas6). Recently, additional Gla proteins have been identified whose function is not well defined to date. Phylloquinone (2-Me-3-polyisoprenyl-1,4-naphthoquinone) from plants and a series of bacterial menaquinones (2-Me-3-polyisoprenyl-1,4-naphthoquinone) are natural forms of the vitamin.

Deficiencies. Historically, vitamin K deficiency has been defined as a disruption of blood clotting due to diminished Gla content of the vitamin K-dependent coagulation factors. Infants are at risk for severe cerebral hemorrhage during the first three to four months after birth, if they do not get enough vitamin K. The reason for vitamin K deficiency in these children is usually impaired fat absorption in conjunction with a low vitamin intake from breastfeeding. (Human milk contains much less vitamin K than infant formulas). In the US and many other countries newborn infants routinely receive vitamin K. Bleeding due to the lack of vitamin K is very rare in older children and adults, presumably, because vitamin K is produced by intestinal bacteria and a small fraction is absorbed from ileum and colon. Oral antibiotic treatment, in conjunction with low vitamin K intake, can induce bleeding. Less than a few days' intake of vitamin K is stored, most of it in liver and bone; in the absence of dietary or intestinal vitamin K sources, symptoms appear rapidly.

Suboptimal vitamin K status which is far more common than outright deficiency may contribute to the progression of osteoporosis and atherosclerosis; research in these areas is promising but preliminary. 4-hydroxy coumarins are vitamin K antagonists that interfere with reactivation of the vitamin and suppress production of mature Gla-proteins needed for coagulation. Some 4-hydroxy coumarins are medically important anticoagulants, others are used as rodenticides.

Diet recommendations. The current Recommended Dietary Allowances (RDAs) for vitamin K (µg/day) are: 5 at age 0-6 months, 10 for 6-12 months, 15 for 1-3 years, 20 for 4-6 years, 30 for 7-10 years, 45 for 11-14 years, 55 for females 15-18 years, 60 for females 19-24 years, 65 for females 25 years and older, pregnant and lactating women and males 15-18; 70 for males 19-24 years, and 80 for males 25 years and older.

Past estimates of vitamin K intake were in the range of a few hundred µg/day; current data suggest that a range of intake of 75-125 µg of phylloquinone is more accurate. Most Americans obtain almost no menaquinones with their diet, but intakes may be very significant for Asians consuming traditional foods. While it is likely that some vitamin K (menaquinones) from bacterial production in the lower intestines is absorbed, the amounts appear to be much less than what is usually available from dietary sources.

Food Sources. Cooked dark green vegetables, such as spinach, kale and broccoli, can provide more than one RDA in a single serving. The bioavailability of vitamin K from different food sources and the effect of food processing is insufficiently known. A small amount of fat is needed for absorption. Natto and similar fermented Asian soy foods also are excellent vitamin K sources. Kiwi, cabbage, liver, soybean, canola and olive oils, including margarine and mayonnaise made from these oils, contain 20-50 % of current RDAs per serving.

Toxicity. Large amounts of phylloquinone or menaquinones can be consumed over extended periods with no toxic effects. Menadione (2-Me-1,4-naphthoquinone) is currently used in animal feeds, but not in foods for human consumption, because it causes hemolytic anemia, hyperbilirubinemia, and kernicterus in infants.

Zinc

Zinc (Zn) is an essential trace mineral. The human body has between 1.5?2.5 g Zn, making it nearly as abundant as iron. It is highly concentrated in specialized areas of the brain, pancreas and adrenal gland, but is present in all cells, particularly in the nucleus. Zinc has structural, catalytic (enzymatic) and regulatory roles. About 1% of the human genome codes for zinc finger proteins, where zinc provides a structural role for regulatory functions. Over 60 enzymes require zinc for activity, including the RNA polymerases. Zinc is actively taken up by synaptic vesicles, supporting a role in neuronal activity and memory. Zinc metabolism is altered during disease and physical stress through hormones, cytokines and toxins, presumably as part of a host defense response.

Deficiencies. An early sign of zinc deficiency in animals is decreased food intake. It is a type II deficiency since a reduction in growth occurs without an apparent reduction in tissue zinc. Reduced immune function, involving B cell and T cell depletion and/or reduced activity, and skin lesions associated with secondary infections are common findings. Chronic zinc deficiency in humans results in reduced growth (dwarfism) and sexual development which are reversible by raising zinc intake. Signs of zinc deficiency may reflect its involvement in cell proliferation and differentiation. Growth, behavioral abnormalities and cognition may respond to zinc supplementation in some populations. Many clinical findings that relate to depressed growth or immunity may have marginal zinc deficiency as a secondary cause.

Clinical uses. Zinc is not widely used as a therapeutic agent except as an ingredient of topical medication. Oral zinc may be used to treat idiopathic skin lesions, some inflammatory conditions and depressed immunity. Zinc is usually indicated in rehabilitation therapy from malnutrition and/or malabsorption in children and adults, used in feeding programs for premature infants and neonates and is also a component of TPN solutions. Supplemental zinc reduces acute diarrhea and depressed immunity.

Diet recommendations. The Recommended Dietary Allowances (RDAs) are: infants, 5 mg/day; children <10 years, 10 mg/day; males >10 years, 15 mg/day; females >10 years, 12 mg/day; pregnancy, 15 mg/day; and lactation, 0-6 mo., 19 mg/day; 7-12 mo., 16 mg/day.

Food sources. Zinc is highly abundant in red and white meat and shellfish. Foods of plant origin except the embryo portion of grains, e.g., wheat germ, are low in zinc. Phytic acid in plants like soybeans binds zinc, forming an insoluble complex that lowers bioavailability. Other inhibitors of absorption are fiber, polyphenols and a high intake of calcium. Zinc from human milk is more absorbable than that from infant formulas or cow's milk.

Toxicity. Acute zinc toxicity is characterized by gastric distress, dizziness and nausea. Symptoms of chronic toxicity include gastric problems, decreased serum ceruloplasmin activity and hypocupremia, decreased lymphocyte stimulation to PHA and reduced HDL cholesterol. An emetic effect occurs at >150 mg Zn/day. Consumption of zinc supplements produces measurable cellular effects but the long term benefit/risk of zinc supplementation has yet to be determined.

18
Dietary Survey

Quantitative information about the food eaten by a people or an community, if compared with physiological standards of human needs, has enabled assessment of nutrition to be made that have been widely used and proved both useful and practical. data can collected covering the whole nation, from families of different economic classes or from individuals of special age groups or occupation.

Each type of survey can provide valuable informatiom.For sound government planning, nation wide data covering all socio economic groups and age groups are required. In all cases the techniques demand care and is time consuming and exacting. Before describing the different methods and their difficulties, certain considerations common to all dietary studies require discussion.

A comparison can be made between the amount of food consumed and a chosen physiological standard only when the data collected have been converted into quantities of energy, carbohydrates, protein, fat, minerals and vitamins. This involves the use of food tables and here errors are inevitably introduced.

Another difficulty is to reach agreement on the physiological or other standards with which to compare the results of dietary surveys. If repeated dietary surveys are carried out systematically in a country, it is possible to tell whether the quantity or quality of the food consumed is improving or declining. This information is often more useful than a comparison with physiological standard, which must always be arbitrary.

National studies—these are attempts to assess the total food supply of a whole nation or other large community. The basic data are the statistics of the imports and exports of foods. In this way it is possible to estimate total food supplies and with a knowledge of the population, to calculate the average daily supply of the principal nutrients.

FAO collected national data on these lines and publishers them at regular intervals. The errors involved in such surveys may be very great. In some countries figures both for agricultural production and population can be nothing more than intelligent guesses. This applies to almost all of Africa and to many Asian and south American countries. On the other hand in a small, Well organized country such as Denmark, the degree of accuracy of such statistics is high.

Another important error that arises in the use of such data is that they give no accurate measure of wastage of foods. FAO usually makes all allowances for losses in the wholesale trade and its figure are intended to describe the food available at the retail or shop level. It is of course, important not to attempt to match such figures directly against a standard of physiological requirements. Some further wastage after purchase is inevitable.

The value of national estimates of food consumption has often been called in question : the errors involved are obvious. Neverthless, an intelligent study of the figures can reveal much that is important about the nutritional status of many countries. Sucessive World food surveys have brought out valuable trends. FAO has done a great service in producing this information, without which the main purpose of the organization could not be achieved—namely the improvement of human nutrition by scientifically planned agriculture.

Family surveys—most surveys have the soldiers, housewives and people in various occupation have been studies. A properly conducted series of individuals dietary surveys gives a good assessment of nutritional status. However, it should never be assumed that an individual is deficient in a nutrient on the basis of a short dietary study. Clinical and biochemical examination are required to confirm any suspicions raised by the intake data.

Short cut methods of estimating dietary intake by recall have been devised. The subject is asked either what he ate the day before or what he eats on a typical day. These methods are subject to inaccuracies but are useful to compare different groups and when repeated, may indicate important trends. The techniques of making individual dietary surveys are described in detailed in along review by Marr (1971) who has given a brief summary of the subject (Marr, 1973).

Comment — the methods of nutritional assessment describe above are of great value in poor communities where evidences of nutrition and mal nutrition is obvious. Dietary and clinical surveys supplemented by a few anthropometric and bio chemical measurements, sufficient to indicate the main order of priorities in a nutritional programme, can be carried out by a small trained staff and at no great expenses. Their value has been proven in many countries in Africa, Asia, Central and South America where the need for their continuing use remains great.

In prosperous countries it is much more difficult to identify and assess small minority groups in whom under nutrition exists. In Britain the committee on Medical Aspects of food policy advises the minister of social security and health on all nutritional problems. They have available the results of the national food survey, the records of school medical services and the tables of mortality given by the registrar general. The national food survey records food consumption in large numbers of homes through out the country each year. As it has been in operation since 1940, it provides material for monitoring changes in patterns of food consumption. However it is not planned primarily to detect the incidence of malnutrition in minority groups. The department of health and social security has carried out nutritional surveys on young children and old people on large scale. These are two groups in which some malnutrition is known to exist, but the surveys have shown that the incidence in both groups is small. In order to detect cases in large numbers of healthy well fed individuals have to be surveyed and large numbers of laboratory tests are required. In consequences the expenses is high. The problem of how to assess quickly the effects of health, if any of a change in national food policy, e.g., the reduction in school milk in 1971, remains unsolved.

In USA the federal Government in 1967 sanctioned a national nutrition survey to determine the prevalence of malnutrition and related health problems among low income population in the United States. Some 40,000 individuals were examined in 10 states and the sample was weighted to include more of the age, income and ethnic groups believed to be at risk of malnutrition. Clinical examination revealed few signs of malnutrition. Anthropometry showed that Negro children were in general taller than whites. Sizeable minorities of children and teenagers were underweight and many adults were obese. The most common positive findings were in the laboratory tests, especially low haemoglobin,which correlated with low dietary or plasma iron, and low plasma vitamin A in Spanish- America, some groups showed biochemical evidence of low intakes of protein, riboflavin and vitamin C. The findings are set out in 940 pages report extending to five books. (US department of health, education and welfare, 1972). This is by far the largest nutrition survey ever carried out.

19
Food Pyramid

The only goal of the Food Guide Pyramid is to give us the best possible advice for healthy eating, then it should be grounded in the evidence and be independent of business.

Instead of waiting for this to happen, nutrition experts from the Harvard School of Public Health created the Healthy Eating Pyramid. It is based on the best available scientific evidence about the links between diet and health. This new pyramid fixes

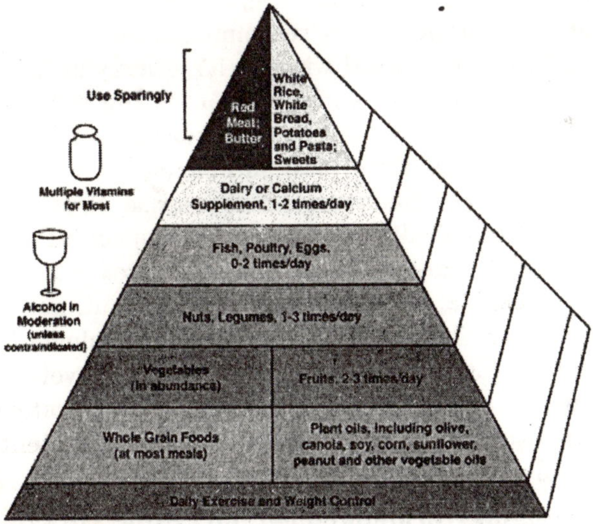

Healthy Eating Pyramid.

fundamental flaws in the USDA pyramid and offers sound information to help people make better choices about what to eat.

The Healthy Eating Pyramid sits on a foundation of daily exercise and weight control. These two related elements strongly influence your chances of staying healthy. They also affect what and how you eat and how your food affects you. The other bricks of the Healthy Eating Pyramid include :

- **Whole Grain Foods (at most meals)**. The body needs carbohydrates mainly for energy. The best sources of carbohydrates are whole grains such as oatmeal, whole-wheat bread, and brown rice. They deliver the outer (bran) and inner (germ) layers along with energy-rich starch. The body can't digest whole grains as quickly as it can highly processed carbohydrates such as white flour. This keeps blood sugar and insulin levels from rising, then falling, too quickly. Better control of blood sugar and insulin can keep hunger at bay and may prevent the development of type 2 diabetes.
- **Plant Oils**. Surprised that the Healthy Eating Pyramid puts some fats near the base, indicating they are okay to eat? Although this recommendation seems to go against conventional wisdom, it's exactly in line with the evidence and with common eating habits. The average American gets one third or more of his or her daily calories from fats, so placing them near the foundation of the pyramid makes sense. Note, though, that it specifically mentions plant oils, not all types of fat. Good sources of healthy unsaturated fats include olive, canola, soy, corn, sunflower, peanut, and other vegetable oils, as well as fatty fish such as salmon. These healthy fats not only improve cholesterol levels (when eaten in place of highly processed carbohydrates) but can also protect the heart from sudden and potentially deadly rhythm problems.(3)
- **Vegetables (in abundance) and Fruits (2 to 3 times)**. A diet rich in fruits and vegetables can decrease the chances of having a heart attack or stroke; protect

against a variety of cancers; lower blood pressure; help you avoid the painful intestinal ailment called diverticulitis; guard against cataract and macular degeneration, the major cause of vision loss among people over age 65; and add variety to your diet and wake up your palate.

- **Fish, Poultry, and Eggs (0 to 2 times)**. These are important sources of protein. A wealth of research suggests that eating fish can reduce the risk of heart disease. Chicken and turkey are also good sources of protein and can be low in saturated fat. Eggs, which have long been demonized because they contain fairly high levels of cholesterol, aren't as bad as they're cracked up to be. In fact, an egg is a much better breakfast than a doughnut cooked in an oil rich in trans fats or a bagel made from refined flour.
- **Nuts and Legumes (1 to 3 times)**. Nuts and legumes are excellent sources of protein, fiber, vitamins, and minerals. Legumes include black beans, navy beans, garbanzos, and other beans that are usually sold dried. Many kinds of nuts contain healthy fats, and packages of some varieties (almonds, walnuts, pecans, peanuts, hazelnuts, and pistachios) can now even carry a label saying they're good for your heart.
- **Dairy or Calcium Supplement (1 to 2 times)**. Building bone and keeping it strong takes calcium, vitamin D, exercise, and a whole lot more. Dairy products have traditionally been Americans' main source of calcium. But there are other healthy ways to get calcium than from milk and cheese, which can contain a lot of saturated fat. Three glasses of whole milk, for example, contains as much saturated fat as 13 strips of cooked bacon. If you enjoy dairy foods, try to stick with no-fat or low-fat products. If you don't like dairy products, calcium supplements offer an easy and inexpensive way to get your daily calcium.
- **Red Meat and Butter (Use Sparingly)** : These sit at the top of the Healthy Eating Pyramid because they contain lots of saturated fat. If you eat red meat every

day, switching to fish or chicken several times a week can improve cholesterol levels. So can switching from butter to olive oil.

- **White Rice, White Bread, Potatoes, Pasta, and Sweets (Use Sparingly)** : Why are these all-American staples at the top, rather than the bottom, of the Healthy Eating Pyramid? They can cause fast and furious increases in blood sugar that can lead to weight gain, diabetes, heart disease, and other chronic disorders. Whole-grain carbohydrates cause slower, steadier increases in blood sugar that don't overwhelm the body's ability to handle this much needed but potentially dangerous nutrient.
- **Multiple Vitamin** : A daily multivitamin, multimineral supplement offers a kind of nutritional backup. While it can't in any way replace healthy eating, or make up for unhealthy eating, it can fill in the nutrient holes that may sometimes affect even the most careful eaters. You don't need an expensive name-brand or designer vitamin. A standard, store-brand, RDA-level one is fine. Look for one that meets the requirements of the USP (U.S. Pharmacopeias), an organization that sets standards for drugs and supplements.
- **Alcohol (in moderation)** : Scores of studies suggest that having an alcoholic drink a day lowers the risk of heart disease. Moderation is clearly important, since alcohol has risks as well as benefits. For men, a good balance point is 1 to 2 drinks a day. For women, it's at most one drink a day.

Bibliography

- USDA/FSIS *Food borne Illness: What Consumers Need To Know*. September 1998.
- Bowlby, J, (1951), maternal care and child health.
- Partnership For Food Safety Education (1997). *Foodborne Illness. A Constant Challenge.*
- Partnership For Food Safety Education (1997). *Four Simple Steps to Fight Back.*
- Angela M. Fraser, Ph.D. Associate Professor/Food Safety Education Specialist and Carolyn J. Lackey, Ph.D. Professor/Food and Nutrition Specialist,North Carolina Cooperative Extension.NC State University, Raleigh, NC 27695-7605.
- *Ball Blue Book*, Alltrista Corporation, Muncie, IN, 1995.
- *Easy to Preserve*, Fourth Edition, Cooperative Extension Service — The University of Georgia, 1999.
- Mock, D.M. (1996) Biotin. In: Present Knowledge in Nutrition (Ziegler, E.E. and Filer, L. J., eds.), 7th ed., pp. 220-235. International Life Sciences Institute Press, Washington, DC.
- Committee on the Scientific Evaluation of Dietary Reference Intakes, Insitute of Medicine. (1998) Dietary Reference Intakes for Thiamin, Riboflavin, Niacin, Vitamin B6, Folate, Vitamin B12, Pantothenic acid, Biotin, and Choline. National Academy Press, Washington, DC.

- Levin, R. J. (1998) In: Modern Nutrition in Health and Disease (Shils, M. E., Olson, J. A., Shike, M. & Ross, A. C., eds.), 9th ed., pp. 49-66. Williams & Wilkins, Baltimore, MD.
- National Research Council. (1989) Diet and Health. Implications for Reducing Chronic Disease Risk. National Academy Press, Washington, DC.
- Rebouche, C. J. (1998) Carnitine. In: Modern Nutrition in Health and Disease (Shils, M. E., Olson, J. A., Shike, M. & Ross, A. C., eds.), 9th ed., pp. 505-512. Williams & Wilkins, Baltimore, MD.
- Grossman, H., Duggan, E., McCamman, S., Welchert, E. & Hellerstein, S. (1980) The dietary chloride deficiency syndrome. Pediatrics 66: 366-374.
- Simopoulos, A. & Bartter, F .C. (1980) The metabolic consequences of chloride deficiency. Nutr. Rev. 38: 201-205.
- Boegehold, M. & Kotchen, T. A. (1991) Importance of dietary chloride for salt sensitivity of blood pressure. Hypertension 17(S1): 158-161.
- Foman, S. J. (1993) Sodium, chloride and potassium. In: Nutrition of Normal Infants (Foman, S.J., ed.), pp. 219-232. Mosby, St. Louis, MO.
- Committee on Nutrition, R. E. Kleinman, ed. Pediatric Nutrition Handbook (1998) American Academy of Pediatrics, Elk Grove Village, IL.
- Anderson, R. A., Cheng, N., Bryden, N. A., Polansky, M. M., Cheng, N., Chi, J. & Feng, J. (1997) Elevated intakes of supplemental chromium improve glucose and insulin variables in individuals with type 2 diabetes. Diabetes 46: 1786-1791.
- Davis, C. M. & Vincent, J. (1997) Chromium oligopeptide activates insulin receptor tyrosine kinase activity. Biochem. 36: 4382-4385.
- Food and Nutrition Board, National Academy of Sciences. (1989) Recommended Dietary Allowances, 10th ed., National Academy Press, Washington, DC.

- Scrimshaw, N. S., Waterlow, J. C. & Schurch, B, eds. (1996) Energy and protein requirements. Eur. J. Clin. Nutr. 50(S1): 1-197.
- Flegal, K. M., Carroll, M. D., Kuczmarski, R. J. & Johnson, C. L. (1998) Overweight and obesity in the United States: prevalence and trends, 1960-1994. Internat. J. Obesity 22: 39-47.
- Bouchard, C., Despres, J. P. & Tremblay, A. (1991) Genetics of obesity and human energy metabolism. Proc. Nutr. Soc. 50: 139-147
- Shils, M. E., Olson, J. A., Shike, M. & Ross, A. C., eds. (1998) Modern Nutrition in Health and Disease, 9th ed., Williams & Wilkins, Baltimore, MD.
- Mauskop, A. & Altura, B. M. (1998) Role of magnesium in the pathogenesis and treatment of migraines. Clin. Neurosci. 5: 24-27.
- Paolisso, G. & Barbagallo, M. (1997) Hypertension, diabetes mellitus, and insulin resistance: the role of intracellular magnesium. Amer. J. Hyperten. 10: 346-355.
- Committee on the Scientific Evaluation of Dietary Reference Intakes, Institute of Medicine (1997) Dietary Reference Intakes for Calcium, Phosphorus, Magnesium, Vitamin D, and Fluoride. National Academy Press, Washington, DC.
- Allen, L. H. & Wood, R. J. (1994) Calcium and phosphorus. In: Modern Nutrition in Health and Disease (Shils, M. E., Olson, J. A. & Shike, M., eds.), 8th ed., pp. 144 - 163. Lea & Febiger, Philadelphia, PA.
- Committee on the Scientific Evaluation of Dietary Reference Intakes (1997) Dietary Reference Intakes: Calcium, Magnesium, Phosphorus, Vitamin D, and Fluoride. National Academy Press, Washington, DC.

Index

Z